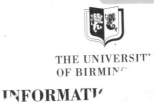

THE UNIVERSIT·
OF BIRMIN·

INFORMATI·

The Biology of Cancer

The Biology of Cancer

The Application of Biology to Cancer Nursing

Edited by

JANICE GABRIEL

MPhil, PgD, BSc(Hons), RGN, FETC, ONC, Cert MHS
Consultant Cancer Nurse, Winchester and
Eastleigh Healthcare NHS Trust/University of Southampton

W

WHURR PUBLISHERS
LONDON AND PHILADELPHIA

© 2004 Whurr Publishers

First Published 2004
Whurr Publishers Ltd
19b Compton Terrace, London N1 2UN, England and
325 Chestnut Street, Philadelphia PA19106, USA

Reprinted 2005

British Library Cataloguing in Publication Data

A catalogue record for this book is available from the
British Library.

ISBN 1 86156 434 1

Printed and bound in the UK by Athenaeum Press Limited,
Gateshead, Tyne & Wear.

Contents

Preface

The application of biology to the delivery of cancer care is playing an increasingly important role in the management of this group of diseases. Although there is a plethora of specialist cancer biology books, they are not aimed at nursing students and practising nurses.

The aim of this book is to be an informative text for students, newly qualified nurses and practising oncology/palliative care nurses. It is also hoped that it will be a useful text for other health-care professionals working in the field of cancer, so that the common questions asked by patients, and their families, can be answered with a clear understanding of the latest advancements in the management of an individual's care.

The aims and objectives of this book are:

- To describe what cancer is, its disease processes and predisposing factors for certain types of malignant conditions.
- To identify the composition of the cell and its functions.
- To discuss the current research that is taking place relating to the biology of cancer.
- To apply research to the management of an individual's disease.
- To summarize current Department of Health guidance applying to care of the individual with cancer.

Janice Gabriel
April 2004

Contributors

David Carpenter, Principal Lecturer, University of Portsmouth

Ailsa Clarke, European Institute of Health and Medical Sciences, University of Surrey

Scott C. Edmunds, Unit of Molecular Pathology, International Agency for Research on Cancer, World Health Organization, Lyon, France.

Guy Gabriel, Translational Oncology Research Centre, University of Portsmouth/Portsmouth Hospitals NHS Trust

Janice Gabriel, Consultant Cancer Nurse, Winchester & Eastleigh Healthcare NHS Trust/University of Southampton

Louise Knight, Translational Oncology Research Centre, University of Portsmouth/Portsmouth Hospitals NHS Trust

Helmout Modjtahedi, Division of Oncology, Post Graduate Medical School, University of Surrey

Carmel Sheppard, Consultant Breast Care Nurse, Portsmouth Hospitals NHS Trust/University of Southampton

Elaine Vickers, Consultant Cancer Nurse, Southampton University Hospitals NHS Trust/University of Southampton

Acknowledgements

I would like to thank the contributors to this book, without whose efforts this work would not have been possible. Despite demanding work schedules, and PhD deadlines in some instances, they kept their promises in meeting deadlines.

I would also like to thank Imogen and Bethany for their understanding. I can at last say 'I have finished my homework'.

JAG

Introduction

This book is written for nurses by experienced, practising health-care professionals to provide a 'readable', comprehensive text that can be easily applied to patient care. The book has not been designed to overwhelm the reader with excessive information on the disease process, but to illustrate how the developments relating to the understanding and application of the biology of cancer can be applied to the management of an individual's disease.

The book is divided into three parts, all of which are evidence based and fully referenced. The first part looks at cancer generally and discusses the disease processes, i.e. the development of a tumour and metastatic spread. It also seeks to identify and explain why there are predisposing factors linked to the development of some cancers.

The second part looks in detail at the cell, its composition, functions and response to cytotoxic agents. It also looks at the roles of the immune system and genetics in relation to the development of malignant disease. This part also deals with the increasing importance in the role of tumour markers in managing a patient's response to treatment.

The final part tackles the area of research. It takes into account the latest research guidelines and applies these to patient care, so that as practising nurses we can have a greater understanding of the potential implications for those of our patients who are considering participation in research studies.

Nurses are playing an increasing role in the management of cancer care. We therefore have a responsibility to our patients to have a sound knowledge base, reflecting the latest research and the application of this research to patient care.

JAG

PART I
UNDERSTANDING CANCER

CHAPTER 1

What is cancer?

JANICE GABRIEL

Cancer is not just one disease, but a generic term used to encompass a group of more than 200 diseases sharing common characteristics. Cancers (carcinomas) are characterized by their unregulated growth and spread of cells to other parts of the body (LeMarbre and Greonwald, 2000). Management of an individual diagnosed with cancer is dependent not only on which type of malignancy they have, but also on the extent of its spread, together with its sensitivity to treatment (Gabriel, 2001).

It is estimated that one in three people in the United Kingdom will develop a malignancy by the time they reach the age of 70, with the incidence increasing with age. This means that about 270 000 individuals receive a cancer diagnosis each year in the UK, with more than 7.5 million affected worldwide (Cornwell, 1997; DoH, 2000a; Corner, 2001). Sadly, the UK incidence of cancer is expected to increase by 2025 (Cornwell, 1997).

This chapter attempts to provide a clearer understanding of what cancers are, and how they spread (metastasize) throughout the body (British Medical Association (BMA), 1997; O'Mary, 2000). It also looks at the importance of staging an individual's disease before determining their most appropriate management (DoH, 2000a, 2000b).

The definition of cancer

As humans we are made up of many millions of cells. Some cells are specific to certain tissues, e.g. epithelial cells are found throughout the gastrointestinal tract, bladder, lungs, vagina, breast and skin. It is this group of cells that accounts for about 70% of cancers (Venitt, 1978; Corner, 2001).

However, any cell has the potential to undergo malignant changes and lead to the development of a carcinoma. The 'tumour' cells are not only confined to localized 'overgrowth' and infiltration of surrounding tissue, but can also spread to other parts of the body via the lymphatic system and bloodstream, creating secondary deposits known as 'metastases' (Walter, 1977; BMA, 1997). The 'normal' cell control mechanisms become disrupted or indeed fail (Corner, 2001). Surgical removal of the original tumour is not always a successful treatment in malignant disease, as a result of microscopic spread. Malignant tumours are often irregular in shape with ill-defined margins (Walter, 1977; Wolfe, 1986). Microscopic spread results in the tissue surrounding the visible tumour appearing unaffected by disease. However, microscopic examination of the surgical resection margins can reveal the presence of malignant cells. If left untreated, these cells will result in localized recurrence of the cancer and eventual spread. The spread of the malignant cells extends outward from the original tumour and has been described as resembling the appearance of a crab. Historically this has been traced back to the origins of the term 'cancer', which was derived from the Latin word for 'crab' (Walter, 1977). Generally, the earlier that a cancer is detected, the less likely it is to metastasize, and so the more favourable the prognosis for the individual.

Metastatic spread

All cells replicate themselves. This is usually about 50–60 times before the cell eventually dies (LeMarbre and Greonwald, 2000; Corner, 2001). However, as malignant cells replicate they grow in an irregular pattern, infiltrating surrounding tissue. This can result in infiltration of the lymphatics and/or blood vessels. By gaining access to these vessels malignant cells can be carried to other sites within the patient's body, where they will replicate and grow, rather like rodents establishing colonies in various parts of a town by gaining access to sewer systems (Walter, 1977; Wolfe, 1986). To ensure that these malignant cells receive nourishment to thrive, angiogenesis occurs, which is the formation of new blood vessels (see Chapter 8) (LeMarbre and Greonwald, 2000).

Lymphatic spread

The malignant cells gain access to the lymphatic system, and travel along the vessels to the 'regional draining' lymph nodes (Walter, 1977). The malignant cell(s) can then establish residency in these regional nodes where they replicate and eventually replace the lymph node with a malignant tumour, i.e. cancer. Malignant cells from this tumour can then spread, via the lymphatic system, to the next group of lymph nodes, thereby spreading the malignancy throughout the patient's body (Walter, 1977). Lymphomas and squamous cell carcinoma of the head and neck commonly spread via the lymphatic system (LeMarbre and Greonwald, 1997).

Blood spread

As with lymphatic spread, malignant cells can also infiltrate the vascular system and travel along the vessels until they arrive at an area where they can become lodged, subsequently replicating to form a secondary (metastatic) deposit. The malignant cells can then migrate via the smaller blood vessels, i.e. the capillaries (Walter, 1977). However, there is evidence to demonstrate that only a small percentage of cells entering the vascular systems actually survive to give rise to blood-borne metastatic spread (Walter, 1977). Malignancies that are linked to blood-borne spread include melanoma and small cell carcinoma of the lung (LeMarbre and Greonwald, 2000).

Liver

The most common site for blood-borne metastases is the liver. Malignancies originating from the gastrointestinal tract, including the pancreas, commonly metastasize to the liver. Other malignancies that can result in secondary deposits in this organ include breast, melanoma, lung and urological cancers (Walter, 1977; Wolfe, 1986).

Lung

The lung is the second most common site for metastatic spread. Tumours that are associated with metastasizing here include breast and stomach cancers, melanomas and sarcomas (Walter, 1977; Wolfe, 1986).

Bone

Bone metastases are commonly associated with malignancies of the breast, prostate, kidney, lung and thyroid. Patients with bone metastases can often present with pain. Pathological fractures are not uncommon as a result of damage of the bone by the malignant cells (Walter, 1977; Wolfe, 1986).

Brain

Brain metastases are closely associated with primary malignancies of the lung, but can also arise from other sites, including the breast and malignant melanoma (Walter, 1977; Wolfe, 1986).

Adrenal glands

Breast and lung primary malignancies are more frequently associated with secondary deposits in the adrenal glands, compared with other sites in the body (Walter, 1977; Wolfe, 1986).

Transcoelomic spread

Transcoelomic spread is the term used to describe invasion of the serosal lining of an organ by malignant cells. The malignant cells trigger an inflammatory response, which results in a serous exudate. It is commonly seen in the peritoneal cavity, where it is associated with ovarian and colonic malignancies (Walter, 1977; Wolfe, 1986).

Staging of malignant disease

To ensure that every patient can be advised about the most appropriate management of his or her particular disease, it is vital that the extent of the cancer is known, e.g. if a patient presents with a breast lump that proves to be malignant, it would be inappropriate to offer the patient a mastectomy if the cancer had already spread to the liver. Removal of the breast would not affect the patient's prognosis, because the cancer would already have metastasized at the time of diagnosis. This is why it is so important to 'stage' a patient's cancer before detailed discussions can take place about the most appropriate treatment option(s).

Most solid tumours, excluding childhood cancers, are 'staged' using the internationally recognized TNM (tumour, node, metastasis) classification system (UICC, 1997). The TNM classification system was introduced into clinical practice in the early 1950s and it aims to ensure that each individual patient is offered the most appropriate treatment for the cancer, depending on the exact extent of the disease. It also provides an indication of the individual's prognosis, by ensuring that health professionals have standardized information when discussing specific cases and their anticipated responses to treatment, e.g. at the patient's pretreatment multidisciplinary meeting (see Chapter 3). By recording this information, future researchers in the treatment of cancer will have a benchmark on which to base assessment of a patient's disease response to potential new treatments (UICC, 1997; O'Mary, 2000).

The TNM classification works by assessing the extent of the primary tumour, the involvement of the lymph glands and the presence of metastases (Table 1.1) (UICC, 1997). A patient diagnosed with a small primary tumour, e.g. T1, will have a more favourable prognosis than a patient with a large primary tumour and widespread metastases.

The staging process will inevitably follow on from the initial diagnostic procedure. This can be a tremendously anxious time for the patient and family members/close friends. The patient has been given a diagnosis of cancer, and will inevitably become concerned about the delay in the start of treatment while waiting for further

Table 1.1 TNM classification system

T = tumour size, e.g.
T0: no evidence of primary tumour
T1, 2, 3, 4: number allocated to size of primary tumour, with '1' representing the
    smallest size, ranging to stage '4'
TX: primary tumour unable to be assessed
N: regional lymph node involvement, e.g.
N0: no evidence of regional lymph involvement
N1, 2, 3, 4: number allocated to involvement of regional lymph nodes ranging
    from '1', confined to one group, up to '4' when several groups are involved
NX: regional lymph nodes unable to be assessed
M = distant metastases, e.g.
M0: no evidence of distant metastatic spread
M1: evidence of distant metastatic spread
MX: distant metastasis cannot be assessed

Note that these are examples only. Not all stages are applicable to some cancers.
From TNM Classification of Malignant Tumours (UICC, 1997).

investigations to determine the stage of the disease. A patient whose staging investigations confirm a small primary cancer confined to his larynx may well be successfully treated with radiotherapy, as opposed to more radical, surgical treatment by laryngectomy. Conversely, a patient with advanced disease that has already metastasized will not have the prognosis improved by undergoing a laryngectomy.

The TNM classification system is commonly used throughout the world for solid tumours, but other classification systems do exist. These include Dukes' staging system for colorectal cancer and Clark's classification for malignant melanoma. For haematological malignancies the TNM classifications are not appropriate because of the systemic nature of the diseases. O'Mary (2000) lists a number of classification systems for haematological malignancies, including the following:

- Ann Arbor classification for lymphomas
- French, American and British (FAB) classifications for myeloblastic leukaemia
- Rai classification for chronic lymphocytic leukaemia.

Diagnostic and staging investigations

Today there are a growing number of tests that can be performed to identify the presence of abnormal cells or an abnormal structure. These tests can initially be undertaken to confirm or eliminate a primary cancer (diagnose), or they can be performed to help in determining the spread of the malignancy (stage). Essentially these investigations fall into three main groups:

- radiology (diagnostic imaging)
- pathology
- endoscopy.

Radiology (diagnostic imaging)

Radiology, or diagnostic imaging, allows for visualization of the internal structures. Images are created that the radiologist then interprets. These images can be created in a number of ways.

X-rays

X-rays or gamma rays are passed through a particular part of the body to generate an image, e.g. a chest radiograph or a mammogram (O'Mary, 2000). To achieve a clearer image, especially in the gastrointestinal tract, lymphatic vessels, urinary tract, etc., contrast medium can be used. This involves injecting or, in the case of gastrointestinal studies, asking the patient to swallow a contrast medium. These contrast media enhance the structures, so providing the clinicians with more detailed information (O'Mary, 2000).

Computed tomography

Computed tomography (CT) is an X-ray technique that involves taking a series of radiographs in 'slices'. The images are then analysed by a computer to produce a three-dimensional picture.

Magnetic resonance imaging

Magnetic resonance imaging (MRI) does not involve the patient or staff being exposed to ionizing radiation. Images are created by the patient lying on a couch within a powerful magnetic field. The magnetic field aligns the patient's hydrogen nuclei, in their cells, in one direction. Pulses of radio waves are used to disturb the magnetized nuclei and change their alignment. This technology results in the generation of images which are captured and analysed by a computer. This procedure is excellent for generating detailed images, especially of soft tissue structures. The procedure from the patient's perspective is not dissimilar to undergoing computed tomography (O'Mary, 2000).

Ultrasonography

Ultrasonography involves the use of high-frequency sound waves. These are directed over a particular area of the patient's body via a probe, resulting in echoes being 'bounced back'. These echoes can then be interpreted to provide information relating to the density of the underlying structures. It is particularly useful in distinguishing cysts from more solid structures (O'Mary, 2000).

Nuclear medicine imaging

This involves the parenteral or enteral administration of radioactive compounds. The radioactive material then concentrates in the organs or tissues under investigation. A special camera (gamma camera) is then used to obtain images of the specific organ/tissues for interpretation by the radiologist.

Positron emission tomography (PET)

Biochemical compounds, 'tagged' with radioactive particles, are administered parenterally to the patient. A special camera is then used to obtain images based on the biochemical and metabolic activity of the tissue (O'Mary, 2000).

Pathology

Pathology tests can be used to confirm a clinical diagnosis and, more recently, to monitor a patient's disease and response to treatment (see Chapters 8 and 9). The types of pathology tests that can be undertaken include the following.

Biochemistry

Body fluids such as blood, urine, etc. can be used to identify values that fall outside the range expected in a 'healthy' individual, e.g. an elevated bilirubin and alkaline phosphatase could be indicative of liver disease. A raised calcium could indicate bone metastases (O'Mary, 2000).

Monoclonal antibodies

The production of monoclonal antibodies can lead to the detection of specific tumour antigens (see Chapter 9).

Tumour markers

These are proteins, antigens, genes or enzymes that can be produced by a tumour. These tests of body fluids, including blood, can be useful in reaching a diagnosis or monitoring an individual's disease (see Chapter 8).

Biopsy

A biopsy provides tissue for histological examination (O'Mary, 1997).

Cytology

This involves looking at cells that have been obtained from fluid, secretions or washings from irrigation of cavities or brushing from tissues (O'Mary, 2000).

Endoscopy

This involves the passage of a long flexible bundle of fibreoptic lights. Images are reflected back to the head of the endoscope to provide the operator with a clear picture of the tissues/organs being viewed. It is possible for the operator to obtain samples of tissue for histological examination. A pair of special forceps is passed through the endoscope to the area requiring biopsy. The tissue is then retrieved through the endoscope and sent to the laboratory. Cells for cytological examination can also be obtained via endoscopic examinations.

Conclusion

Cancer is a complex group of diseases, which currently affect one in three of those living in the UK. Successful treatment is dependent not only on advances in medical science, but also on the earlier detection of disease and careful staging to determine the extent of the cancer at the time of diagnosis.

CHAPTER 2

Predisposing factors to developing cancer

JANICE GABRIEL

As society becomes more affluent, so the incidence of cancer can be demonstrated to rise. There could be a number of explanations for this, including increased wealth and improved health care enabling individuals to achieve a greater life expectancy than their grandparents (Gabriel, 2001). People are also surviving previously life-threatening illnesses, such as infectious diseases, major accidents, etc., only to live longer and possibly to develop cancer later in life. We also know that more affluent societies consume higher amounts of convenience foods, alcohol and tobacco, as well as being exposed to higher levels of chemicals and pollutants compared with people living in some less developed parts of the world. All these factors can contribute to an individual developing a malignancy (Venitt, 1978; Cartmel and Reid, 2000; Corner, 2001). Other factors can include past exposure to ionizing radiation, viruses and a genetic disposition (Cartmel and Reid, 2000; Yarbro, 2000a).

This chapter looks at the possible links between specific cancers and the lifestyles that people adopt, together with the environments in which they live. It will also identify the steps that are being taken to minimize the risks and to identify cancers at an earlier stage.

Historical perspective

As long ago as 1775, Percival Pot, a London surgeon, described the link between cancer of the scrotum and chimney sweeps' boys (Walter, 1977). Pot observed that there was a higher incidence of carcinoma of the scrotum in boys who worked sweeping chimneys than those employed in other occupations. Although not designed as a scientific study to establish the cause of cancer in this group of boys, a causal link was identified. Horton-Taylor (2001) writes about the study undertaken by Doll and Hill, in the 1950s, looking

11

at the incidence of lung cancer among British doctors. This study established a link between smoking and the development of small cell (oat cell) carcinoma of the lung. Further work undertaken by Doll and Hill has identified that the risk of dying from lung cancer is 32 times higher in heavy smokers compared with non-smokers (Horton-Taylor, 2001). A laboratory experiment, undertaken in 1915, proved for the first time that it was possible to develop cancer as a direct result of exposure to a chemical – coal tar. It was applied directly to the skin of a rabbit, resulting in the development of skin cancer (Yarbro, 2000a). In 1896 a German physicist, Roentgen, identified the use of radiation (X-rays) as a diagnostic tool. Further work looking at the use of radiation resulted in it being used as a new treatment for cancer by the close of the nineteenth century. However, within 7 years of Roentgen discovering the use of X-rays as a diagnostic tool, a causal link between exposure to radiation and the development of leukaemia was established (Yarbro, 2000a).

At the beginning of the twenty-first century we have come a long way since Pot's chance observation identifying the cause of cancer of the scrotum in chimney sweeps' boys – the earliest described occupationally acquired malignancy. Studies are now undertaken specifically to identify whether there are causal links between exposure to certain substances and the development of cancer.

Diet

Colorectal cancer

Back in 1978 Gillis and Holes highlighted a link between a low-fibre diet and carcinoma of the large bowel (Gillis, 1978). Today it is well recognized that a diet low in fibre and high in animal fats can significantly contribute to the development of colorectal cancer (Cartmel and Reid, 2000; Yarbro, 2000b). The consumption of five portions of fresh fruit and vegetables each day is believed to decrease the risk factors of developing this type of malignancy (Department of Health (DoH), 2000a). *The NHS Cancer Plan* (DoH, 2000a) advocates increasing the daily consumption of fresh fruit and vegetables to reduce the risk of developing cancer in later life.

It is estimated that a third of all cancers are directly linked to diet and possibly as many as 90% of colorectal malignancies (Yarbro, 2000b). In the UK, 25000 individuals are diagnosed with colorectal cancer each year and the incidence is increasing (Harrocopus and Myers, 1996). Most of those affected by this disease, i.e. 75%, will be older than 65 years, with a median age of 70 (Cartmel and Reid, 2000).

Incidence of colorectal cancer in the UK (Whittaker and Sheppard, 2001)

- Under 50 years: 4 per 100 000
- In 50–69 year olds: 100 per 100 000
- In people aged over 70: 300 per 100 000.

Breast cancer

The development of cancer, linked to dietary factors, is not solely confined to colorectal malignancies. In 1975, a study by Armstrong and Doll identified a diet high in fats as a possible contributing cause to the development of breast cancer (Willett, 1989; Sheppard 2001). However, Yarbro (2000b) suggests that the consumption of fat alone is not a possible contributing cause, but rather the total number of calories, especially the calories consumed in early life.

Stomach cancer

In Japan there is a high incidence of stomach cancer, which is far more common than other types of malignancies in that country. Yet, when Japanese people have moved to the USA, it has been observed that the incidence of stomach cancer reduces and the incidence of breast and colorectal malignancies increases in line with the indigenous population. This has been highlighted by Willett (1989) as being directly explained by change in diet, i.e. the Japanese have abandoned/reduced their former diets, which contained high amounts of salted fish, in favour of a more western diet that is high in fat and low in fibre.

Tobacco/smoking

There is overwhelming evidence to link tobacco with a variety of cancers. Although smoking unquestionably contributes significantly to the development of small cell (oat cell) carcinoma of the lung and bladder cancer, it must not be forgotten that tobacco can be consumed in a variety of different ways (Cartmel and Reid, 2000). These can include chewing, sniffing and inhalation from passive smoking. The malignant conditions linked to the use of/exposure to tobacco can include the following (Horton-Taylor, 2001):

- small cell (oat cell) carcinoma of the lung
- oropharyngeal cancer
- bladder cancer
- cervical cancer
- gastric cancer

- lip cancer
- pancreatic cancer.

Lung cancer

Lung cancer is now one of the most common malignancies affecting both men and women in the UK (Horton-Taylor, 2001). Although its incidence is decreasing in males, it is still rising in the female population (Gillis, 1978). This is not a pattern unique to the UK, because the incidence of smoking-related lung cancers is not expected to peak among American women until 2010 (Cartmel and Reid, 2000). Studies in both the USA and the UK indicate that, despite the publicity linked to cigarette smoking and cancer, the incidence is continuing to rise, especially in females from lower socioeconomic groups (Gillis, 1978; Cartmel and Reid, 2000). The government is well aware of the huge part that smoking plays in the development of cancers. *The NHS Cancer Plan* (DoH, 2000a) aims to reduce smoking in adults, from 28% to 24% by 2010, by developing local targeted action. This includes the provision of services to help individuals quit smoking and the availability of nicotine replacement therapy on prescription from April of 2001 (DoH, 2001a).

Passive smoking

Passive smoking is also linked to the development of cancer among non-smokers. There have been a number of litigation cases in the USA, where compensation has been paid to individuals diagnosed with smoking-related malignancies, who have involuntarily shared office space with smokers for many years (Fielding and Phenow, 1998).

Oral cancer

In India cancer of the oral cavity accounts for a high percentage of all malignancies registered annually. This malignancy is linked to the social habit of chewing quids of betel, lime and tobacco. The constant irritation to the tissues of the cheek and gum can lead over time to the individual developing an oral malignancy (Gillis, 1978).

Bladder cancer

Smoking was first linked to the development of bladder cancer in the mid-1950s (Lind and Hagan, 2000). Studies have identified that as many as 50% of cases of bladder cancer could be directly attributable to smoking (Gillis, 1978; Lind and Hagan, 2000).

Viruses

Early work looking at the link between viruses and the development of cancers has led to the discovery of human genes associated with cancer (Yarbro, 2000b). Probably the most common malignancy linked to viral exposure is that of hepatitis B in liver cancer (Hausen, 1991; Yarbro, 2000b). However, there are a number of other viruses linked to specific cancers, including:

- HTLV-1: T-cell lymphoma and T-cell leukaemia
- HTLV-2: hairy-cell leukaemia
- Epstein–Barr virus: Burkitt's lymphoma
- Hepatitis B virus: liver cancer
- Hepatitis C virus: liver cancer
- Human papilloma virus: cervical cancer.

Bacteria

Helicobacter pylori can live in the lining of the stomach and is linked to the development of gastric and duodenal ulcers. It is now known that there is a link between chronic ulcer disease and the development of malignancy. This bacterium can be eradicated by treatment with antibiotics, therefore reducing the risk to the individual of developing gastric cancer in the future (Yarbro, 2000b).

Radiation

Today it is well recognized that exposure to radiation can have a carcinogenic effect on living cells. Ionizing radiation releases enough energy to damage the DNA within each cell, which can result in malignant changes taking place in later life. Exposure can be in the form of repeated doses or in one isolated incident (Walter, 1977; Yarbro, 2000b).

The most common forms of radiation-induced cancers are basal cell carcinoma and squamous carcinoma of the skin. These forms of malignancy can arise from excessive exposure to ultraviolet radiation (UVR), i.e. the sun (Cartmel and Reid, 2000).

The use of radiation in medicine and industry is now closely controlled, with the specified maximum annual dose for each individual closely monitored (Palmer, 2001). Over time and with increasing knowledge of the potential dangers of ionizing radiation, these annual doses have been reduced (Palmer, 2001). Exposure to ionizing radiation can result in the following malignancies:

- Leukaemia
- Thyroid cancer
- Squamous cell carcinoma of the skin.

Asbestos

Exposure to asbestos is now known to be responsible for the malignancy known as mesothelioma. Up until the 1970s asbestos was widely used in the UK building industry. The asbestos, in the form of a fine, white powder, was inhaled by the staff who handled the material. The onset of the resulting malignancy, i.e. mesothelioma, could run over a period of many years from the initial exposure. The use of asbestos has now been greatly reduced. When it is handled, e.g. in the demolition of buildings, staff exposure is closely monitored with strict enforcement in the provision of protective clothing (Cartmel and Reid, 2000; Yarbro, 2000b).

Chemicals

Today it is well recognized that a number of chemicals, if not handled correctly, can be linked to the development of cancer in later life (these are summarized in Table 2.1). Where occupational exposure is unavoidable, legislation exists to ensure that exposure is minimized and the health of individuals is closely monitored (Cartmel and Reid, 2000; Yarbro, 2000b).

Table 2.1 Chemicals/agents linked to specific cancers

Chemical/agent	Cancer type
Asbestos	Mesothelioma
Pitch, soot, coal tar, oil	Squamous cell carcinoma of the skin, scrotum
Vinyl chloride	Liver
Arsenic	Sinuses, lung
Benzidine	Bladder
Wool/leather/wood dust	Nasal sinuses
Aniline dyes	Bladder

Pollution

As our society becomes more affluent, so we consume more and generate increasing waste products, which can lead to pollution. Our increasing use of chlorofluorocarbons (CFCs) has led to the partial destruction of the ozone layer, resulting in more ultraviolet radiation reaching the earth. This is believed to be a contributing factor to the increase in the number of skin cancers, so steps are being taken to reduce the amount of CFCs in use, e.g. seeking alternatives to 'spray' containers for products.

Genetics

With the development of molecular biology, new techniques are leading to the identification of genes that can increase an individual's risk of cancer. Genes already identified include those shown in Table 2.2.

It is believed that as many as 15% of all cancers have a genetic link (Lynch and Alban, 1984; Yarbro, 2000a). However, with advances in medical science, including the Human Genome Project, this estimate could be revised as new knowledge is acquired. We already know that the damage to genes, by such substances as tobacco, radiation, etc. can lead to gene mutation. These damaged (mutated) genes then go on to develop cancer, if their replication is unchecked (see Chapter 6).

Table 2.2 Genes and associated cancer

Gene	Associated cancer
RB1	Retinoblastoma
WT1	Wilms' tumour
APC	Familial polyposis
CDKN2	Dysplastic naevus syndrome
FACC	Fanconi's anaemia
BLM	Bloom syndrome (associated with leukaemia)
BRCA-1	Breast and ovarian cancer
BRCA-2	Breast cancer

From Yarbro (2000b).

The NHS Cancer Plan

In September 2000 *The NHS Cancer Plan* was published by the Department of Health (2000a). This publication has four main aims. These are:

- to save more lives
- to ensure that people with cancer get the right professional support and care as well as the best treatments
- to tackle the inequalities in health that mean unskilled workers are twice as likely to die from cancer as professionals
- to build for the future through investment in the cancer workforce, through strong research and through preparation for the genetics revolution, so that the NHS never falls behind in cancer care again.

This document identifies the government's strategy for tackling cancer. Not only has cancer been made one of the main priorities within the NHS; for the first time a cohesive approach to care will be employed throughout the entire patient journey. Primary, secondary and tertiary care will work with the voluntary sector and consumers of health care, i.e. patients and carers, to develop effective programmes for prevention, diagnosis, treatment, care and research (DoH, 2000a). *The NHS Cancer Plan* (DoH, 2000a) has set out clear objectives for providers of cancer services to meet, to ensure that all patients have access to speedier diagnostic services and treatment. By 2001 all patients who are suspected of having a possible cancer, when they consult their general practitioner, are referred to the appropriate hospital specialist and seen within 2 weeks. Hospitals are required to monitor these referrals to ensure that, if breaches in the waiting times do occur, appropriate action can be taken to rectify the problem. By 2005 no patient will be expected to wait more than 2 months (62 days) from urgent referral by their general practitioner to treatment (DoH, 2000a).

Health promotion

The development of cancers can be a result of lifestyles adopted over many years. Health promotion needs to start at an early age in order to have a maximum effect in reducing an individual's risk of developing cancer in later life. It has already been discussed that as many as a third of all cancers are linked to diet, with a further third linked to smoking (Cartmel and Reid, 2000; Yarbro, 2000b). By working closely with health promotion departments and primary care, the government intends to continue to reduce the incidence of smoking. This is to be achieved by (DoH, 2000a):

- banning tobacco advertising
- developing NHS-provided smoking cessation services
- providing nicotine replacement therapy on prescription
- enforcing the law to prohibit the sale of cigarettes to children under 16
- establishing a smoking cessation helpline.

To raise the awareness of the importance of the consumption of fresh fruit and vegetables, the government is committed to working closely with the food industry and the Food Standards Agency (DoH, 2000a). The overall intention is to increase the availability and affordability of fresh fruit and vegetables to all members of society, with a recommendation that at least five pieces/portions should be consumed each day. One initiative includes 'The National School Fruit Scheme', which will ensure that all children aged between 4 and 6 will receive a free piece of fruit each day at school (DoH, 2000a).

Other areas that are being addressed through health promotion campaigns include raising the awareness of heavy alcohol consumption linked to the development of cancer, the dangers of inappropriate protection from sunlight, reducing obesity and the importance of regular physical activity (DoH, 2000a).

Health screening

It is important to understand the difference between 'screening' and 'testing'. Screening is intended to look at large numbers of asymptomatic individuals in an attempt to identify a potential underlying problem at an early stage. Testing is a specific intention to find out the cause of an individual's symptoms. Individuals included in screening programmes tend to have generalized characteristics, e.g. they fall into a specific age band or are of the same sex, e.g. by 2004 all women aged between 50 and 70 will be included in the national breast screening programme (DoH, 2000a). Screening investigations should be minimally invasive and not too uncomfortable, in order to ensure maximum take-up by the target population. A diagnostic test is a deliberate attempt to identify the cause of an individual's symptoms. If someone has a positive screening result he or she will inevitably be advised to undergo further investigations. In such cases more invasive, diagnostic tests may well be suggested to determine the cause of the abnormality (Gabriel, 2001).

Breast screening

The breast-screening programme was launched in the UK in 1988. All women aged between 50 and 64 were invited to undergo breast screening mammography every 3 years. By 2004 this programme will be extended to include all women aged between 50 and 70 and include two radiographs of each breast (DoH, 2000a).

Cervical screening

In 1988 a national cervical screening programme was established in the UK for all women aged between 20 and 64. Since its introduction the death rate from cervical cancer has been reducing year on year (DoH, 2000a).

Prostate screening

Some men diagnosed with prostate cancer have elevated levels of prostate-specific antigen (PSA). There is also a percentage of men with an elevated PSA who do not have prostate cancer. As yet there is not enough knowledge about the possible links between an elevated PSA and prostate cancer to enable a screening programme to be developed based on the PSA blood test alone. There is currently ongoing research in this area (see Chapter 8).

Colorectal screening

There is strong evidence to link the early detection and treatment of colorectal cancer to improved survival rates. A pilot study is currently being undertaken to ascertain whether screening, using the faecal occult blood test, is not only acceptable to patients, but also effective in detecting bowel cancer at an earlier stage (DoH, 2000a).

Research is also being undertaken to evaluate the effectiveness of flexible sigmoidoscopy in screening for colorectal cancers (DoH, 2000a).

Ovarian screening

Currently two possible techniques are being looked at as potential screening methods for ovarian cancer. These include transvaginal ultrasonography and a blood test for the antigen CA125 (see Chapter 8) (DoH, 2000a).

Early detection

Although a reduction in the risks associated with the development of cancer plays a key role in reducing the overall incidence of the disease, the next biggest challenge is to be able to identify the disease at an earlier stage. Improvements in diagnostic imaging and pathology unquestionably play vital roles here. We have already touched on the advances in medical research leading to the identification of specific tumour markers (see Chapter 8), but we need to raise the awareness of health professionals and members of the public. Through the publication of *The NHS Cancer Plan* (DoH, 2000a), hospitals have issued guidance, on the referral criteria, to GPs for patients with clinical features that could be suggestive of an underlying malignancy. Patients referred under this mechanism are now fast tracked to see an appropriate specialist. They are then prioritized to undergo diagnostic tests to ensure that a diagnosis is reached without any inappropriate delays. As a result of the publicity surrounding the publication of *The NHS Cancer Plan* (DoH, 2000a) many more individuals are aware of what the early signs of cancer could be, resulting in more patients consulting their GPs.

Conclusion

The incidence of cancer is increasing for a variety of reasons: lifestyles, increasing age of the population, etc. However, more streamlined approaches to care, especially in relation to health promotion, early detection and prompt treatment, should ultimately see a decrease in the overall mortality associated with this group of diseases. The benefits of research will not only be beneficial to those affected by the disease, but also will have implications for society as a whole. New genetic tests and future research will, it is hoped, be able to influence the development of cancer for future generations.

CHAPTER 3

Cancer: what does a diagnosis mean for an individual and what are the implications for society?

JANICE GABRIEL

Every year in the United Kingdom about 270 000 individuals are diagnosed with cancer, with a further 120 000 dying in England alone as a direct result of this group of diseases (Cornwell, 1997; Department of Health (DoH), 2000a). It is currently estimated that one in three people in the UK will develop a malignancy by the age of 70. This equates to 700 individuals each day, in England, receiving a diagnosis of cancer (DoH, 2000a).

This chapter attempts to discuss some of the issues that a diagnosis of cancer can raise for an individual and his or her family. It also outlines the government's efforts to improve the standard of cancer services, and what this means for patients embarking on their 'cancer journey'.

A diagnosis of cancer

> Volumes are now written and spoken upon the effects of the mind on the body. Much of it is true. But I wish a little more was thought of the effect of the body on the mind
>> Florence Nightingale (1859 – cited in Price, 1990, p. xii)

Almost 150 years have passed since Florence Nightingale wrote these words. Cancer is a protracted illness, always raising uncertainty in the minds of those affected, and their families, as to whether the disease can be successfully treated. Historically, the management of an individual with cancer has revolved around medical models, which are investigation, diagnosis, treatment and follow-up. Although some efforts have been made in the past in addressing the holistic needs of patients and their families, it is only recently that there has been national guidance, resulting in national standards, which are contained in the *Manual of Cancer Standards* (DoH, 2000a, 2000b; Whittaker and Sheppard, 2001; Young, 2001).

As discussed earlier in this book, cancer is a group of diseases, with some forms of malignancy, such as basal cell carcinoma of the skin, carrying an excellent prognosis for the patient (Ketcham and Loescher, 2000). However, the word 'cancer' has been used. As health professionals we must not be complacent when using the word 'cancer'. It is important that the diagnosis is imparted to the patient, and their families and carers, with tact and adequate explanation of its potential implications, even if it is a form of the disease that responds well to treatment (DoH, 2000a; Young, 2001). Cancer instils fear in most individuals affected. Many patients, together with their family and friends, experience feelings of uncertainty about their future. Young (2001) discusses how patients want honest and positive answers. Is the disease treatable? If so, what will the treatment involve – surgery, radiotherapy, chemotherapy? What is the likelihood of the success of the treatment? Will the cancer, or indeed the treatment, result in any adverse effects in the future? What is the risk of the cancer returning? Is there any inherited risk with this type of cancer? If the cancer is untreatable, what can be done? What does the future hold? What are the financial implications for the individual and the family? Will the cancer affect the relationship between the patient and his or her partner? We all find bad news distressing, but how we react depends on our personalities and circumstances. Young (2001) discusses how some individuals experience the 'grief' process at different stages, e.g. when they embark on the investigation trail for a possible diagnosis of cancer, or when they are given the diagnosis of cancer. It is not only the patient who requires time and support, but also their family and friends for the entire patient journey – a journey that is unique for every individual and carer (DoH, 2000a).

The NHS Cancer Plan (DoH, 2000a) stresses the importance of good communication between health professionals and patients. But, however good communication is, it alone is inadequate. The individual patient, together with carer(s) and family members, needs the offer of ongoing support from the time of diagnosis and throughout the entire patient journey. If the 'offer' is initially refused, health professionals need to ensure that it is repeated at appropriate times. Support can take the form of 'active listening', providing written information, or onward referral to other professionals, such as specialist nurses, social workers, palliative care specialists, counselling services, voluntary organizations, etc. Whatever support is offered, it must be appropriate for that individual (Young, 2001).

The NHS Cancer Plan (DoH, 2000a) summarizes some surveys of cancer patients, identifying that patients give great importance to:

- Being treated with humanity – with dignity and respect
- Good communication with health professionals
- Being given clear information about their condition
- Receiving the best possible symptom control
- Receiving psychological support when they need it

DoH (2000a, p. 64)

Each patient is a unique individual, and as such we as health professionals must respond to their individual requirements, irrespective of their social, cultural, religious background, etc. We should not raise unrealistic expectations, but at the same time we must be honest, yet sensitive to the content of our discussions. For most patients they are embarking on a long and complex journey – a journey for which no one can guarantee the outcome, a journey that is unique to them.

The NHS Cancer Plan

Back in 1995 a document was published by the Department of Health known as *A Framework for Commissioning Cancer Services* (DoH, 1995), commonly referred to as the Calman–Hine report. This document recommended the establishment of specialist cancer networks in England and Wales, and these networks would be responsible for coordinating the care provided in primary, secondary and tertiary care, to ensure that all individuals receive equity of access and a uniformly high standard of cancer care, delivered by a skilled and knowledgeable cancer workforce. Today there are 34 cancer networks in England.

Following on from the publication of the Calman–Hine report (DoH, 1995), *The NHS Cancer Plan* (DoH, 2000a) was published in the autumn of 2000. This document stated four aims which are given in Chapter 2, page 17.

The NHS Cancer Plan (DoH, 2000a) is an ambitious document setting out a strategy to integrate the prevention, screening, diagnosis, treatment and ongoing care for individuals. It also acknowledges that, to achieve its aims, significant investment is required, not only in the provision of new and replacement equipment, but also in specialist and improved staffing, information systems and drugs. At the heart of the plan is the patient. To ensure that health professionals take into account the views of 'users' of their services, cancer networks are expected to work with patients, carers and voluntary groups, to take into account their views for the future provision of cancer services.

After the publication of *The NHS Cancer Plan* (DoH, 2000a), there were over 65 000 responses to a national questionnaire, seeking patients' views on the provision of NHS cancer services, before July 2002 (DoH, 2002). The respondents to this questionnaire identified that there could be improvement in the provision of information relating to their diagnosis and treatment, together with the support and time available from health professionals (DoH, 2002).

Many of the cancer networks are working with the voluntary organization CancerVOICES. CancerVOICES is a national project, working with individuals affected by cancer, together with other groups involved in providing support for patients and carers. One of the aims of the project is to encourage those who have experience of cancer services to share their experiences and influence the future provision of cancer care (CancerVOICES, 2002). Groups, linked to their local cancer network, are actively working with health professionals on a range of projects, including the development of information materials, development of guidelines, participation in multiprofessional network groups, etc. (CancerVOICES, 2002).

Successful treatment for cancer depends very much on how early an individual patient presents and is diagnosed. Before the publication of *The NHS Cancer Plan* (DoH, 2000a), a 'fast-track' referral system was being implemented throughout the country for all patients visiting their general practitioner with clinical features suggestive of cancer. As a result, by December 2000, a 'roll-out' programme has meant that all patients with a suspected cancer should wait no longer than 2 weeks from the time of referral by their GP until they see a specialist (DoH, 2000a). By 2005 no patient will wait longer than a month (31 days) from diagnosis to treatment, and no more than 2 months (62 days) from urgent GP referral to treatment (DoH, 2000a).

Faster access to diagnosis does not necessarily mean that all patients can currently benefit from speedier treatment. Insufficient staff means not only that an investment in the future workforce is required, but also that a coordinated approach is needed, questioning who is the most appropriate group of health professionals to undertake specific tasks/roles. Training of future staff needs to go hand in hand with ongoing career development. This will ensure not only that individual health professionals can realize their full potential, but also that patients can benefit from timely and appropriate care from a skilled and knowledgeable health professional. Individual Trusts are working with their cancer network and Workforce Development Confederation (WDC) to develop strategies to meet these challenges (DoH, 2000a).

Cancer Services Collaborative

The Cancer Services Collaborative (CSC) is part of the NHS Modernization Agency. The objective of the CSC teams, which are linked to individual networks, is to look at the provision of specific cancer services within an organization, e.g. breast cancer, and 'map' the patient journey. The results of this mapping exercise identify where the delays are for the patient. Before the publication of *The NHS Cancer Plan* (DoH, 2000a), nine cancer networks were already taking part in CSC projects. The results from these early projects clearly highlighted that many of the delays in patients' treatment were a result of the way the 'systems' for delivering their care were organized. Through working with all the staff involved, the 'systems' could be redesigned to expedite patients' journeys, e.g. pre-booking patients at the time of referral for diagnostic tests, based on the information contained in their referral letter (DoH, 2000a).

The patient journey

Most patients will initially consult their GPs before embarking on their 'patient journey'. If their GP considers that they have clinical features that could be suggestive of an underlying malignancy, they will be referred to an appropriate specialist under the 'rapid access' criteria (DoH, 2000a, 2000b). However, a small percentage of patients may well present as an emergency, e.g. with an obstructed bowel, or as a result of 'routine' investigations for symptoms not believed to be related to an underlying malignancy. Whatever route the patient takes, it is essential that a diagnosis is made and the extent (stage) of the cancer determined before the patient can be advised on what is the most appropriate treatment (see Chapter 1). In accordance with the *Manual of Cancer Standards* (DoH, 2000b) all patients should have their management discussed at a multidisciplinary team meeting, e.g. this means that to comply with the *Manual of Cancer Standards* (DoH, 2000b, p. 44) a breast multidisciplinary team should consist of the following 'core' members:

- Designated breast surgeon
- Breast care nurse(s)
- Radiologist
- Histopathologist
- Oncologist.

In addition to the above, the 'core' team should have access to the following individuals who are known as 'extended team' members (DoH, 2000b, p. 49):

- Palliative care team member
- Breast radiographer
- Psychiatrist or clinical psychologist
- Social worker
- Plastic/reconstructive surgeon
- Clinical geneticist/genetic counsellor
- Physiotherapist/lymphoedema specialist.

Such discussions should ensure that every patient is advised about the most appropriate management by health professionals who are experienced and knowledgeable about the specific cancer. These discussions also ensure that individual patients can benefit from a holistic approach to their care, with support from the site-specific clinical nurse specialist, and early onward referral to other members of the team, such as physiotherapist, palliative care team, etc., as appropriate. A typical patient journey is depicted in Figure 3.1.

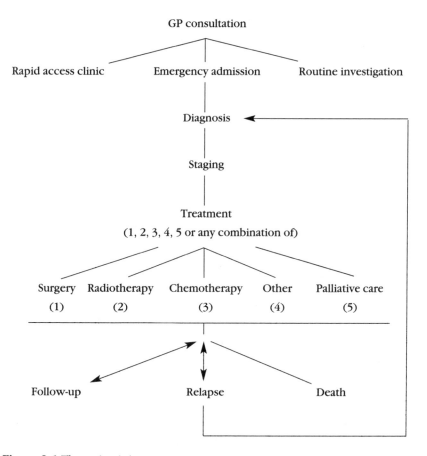

Figure 3.1 The patient's journey.

The impact of research on patient care

The NHS Cancer Plan (DoH, 2000a) highlights the importance of research for the detection and treatment of cancer. In particular it highlights the importance of research into the genetic and cellular changes that lead to an individual developing cancer. The Plan states (DoH, 2000a, p. 91):

> 10.26 The genetic makeup of an individual may determine how effective a particular medicine is and the risk of adverse side effects. Research in this area, known as pharmacogenetics, is accelerating as a result of the Human Genome Project. Genes affecting the metabolism of more than twenty drugs, including anti-cancer agents, have been identified.
>
> 10.27 In the future, successful chemotherapy is likely to become increasingly dependent on understanding an individual's genetic background. In partnership with other cancer research funders, we will promote the development of pharmacogenetic studies in the area of cancer chemotherapy.

As health-care professionals we must ensure that every patient has the opportunity to benefit from the latest research and, where appropriate, be offered the opportunity to participate in a clinical trial if it is considered appropriate for his or her individual circumstances. *The NHS Cancer Plan* (DoH, 2000a) states that a review undertaken by the Department of Health in 1999 considers support for research into cancer as a high priority. This has resulted in the establishment of the National Cancer Research Network (NCRN) in April 2001 (*NCNR Newsletter*, November 2001). The aim of the NCRN is to increase the activity and quality of cancer research in the UK. This has resulted in the establishment of research networks, which are linked closely with the 34 cancer networks. Over a 3-year period, which is by 2004, the NCRN is aiming to double the number of individual patients recruited into trials. Professor Selby (Director of NCRN), writing in the first issue of the *NCRN Newsletter* (November 2001), stated that cancer research would be strengthened by the creation of two additional groups: the National Translational Cancer Research Network (NTRAC) and the National Cancer Research Institute (NCRI). He went on to explain that the NCRI represented the main funders of cancer research, and that NTRAC would be concentrating on the initial development of translational research (see Chapter 10).

Conclusion

Although cancer is a common group of diseases, affecting more than a quarter of a million people in the UK every year, each patient is an individual, and every patient requires information and support pertaining to his or her individual needs, at the various stages of his or her journey.

Cancer also has an impact on the patient's family and friends. They too require information and support, throughout the whole patient journey and beyond, when treatment options have been exhausted. Patients and carers should be involved in working with health professionals, to identify the information and support that are required.

As health professionals we need to adopt a team approach. We need to work with our patients and their carers to ensure that they not only receive evidence-based care, but also have the opportunity to participate in clinical trials, if it is appropriate for their individual circumstances.

The chapters in this book should help health professionals gain a greater understanding of the research that is taking place to apply the biology of cancer to direct patient care.

PART II
THE SCIENCE OF CANCER

CHAPTER 4
The cell

LOUISE ALICE KNIGHT

The human body is made up of about 10 trillion cells, and the ability of each of these to produce exact replicas is an essential component of life. To begin to understand how things might go wrong and cancer may develop, it is essential to understand normal cellular processes.

What is a cell?

The cell is the basic unit of all living matter, whether it is a single-celled bacterium such as *Escherichia coli* or a multicelled organism such as a human being.

Every cell is remarkable; not only does it have the ability to carry out complex tasks, e.g. uptake of nutrients and conversion to energy and the ability to replicate, but it also contains all the instructions to carry out these tasks. Cells are divided into two types: (1) prokaryotes and (2) eukaryotes.

Prokaryotes lack a nuclear membrane (the membrane that surrounds the nucleus) and the best-known examples of prokaryotic organisms are bacteria. They are made up of a cell envelope within which is found the cytoplasmic region, which contains cytoplasm – a fluid made up of about 70% water, with the remainder consisting of enzymes that the cell has manufactured, amino acids, glucose molecules and adenosine triphosphate (ATP). At the centre of the cell is its DNA, which as a result of the lack of a nuclear membrane floats within the cytoplasm.

In comparison, eukaryotes contain cell organelles; similar to organs within the body, each organelle has its own structure and specific function or metabolic process to carry out. Figure 4.1 illustrates some of the organelles that are found within the eukaryotic cell; among these is the nucleus, which is composed of three main parts:

1. Nucleolus: this is the most prominent part of the nucleus and its function is to produce ribosomes.

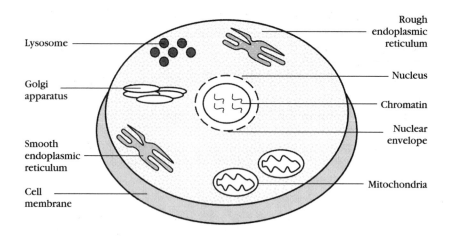

Figure 4.1 A typical eukaryotic cell and some of the components that are found within it.

2. Nuclear envelope: this is a double-layered membrane, which protects and separates the nucleus from the cytoplasm and molecules that could cause damage.
3. Chromatin: this is a DNA–protein complex containing our genes; during replication it condenses into chromosomes.

It is the nucleus that gives the eukaryote (meaning 'true nucleus') its name.

Other important components that are illustrated in Figure 4.1 include the following:

- Cell membrane: this is made up of a double layer of lipid molecules, which gives the cell support and protection, letting nutrients in and waste molecules out. It is able to alter its shape and receive signals from the outside environment.
- Mitochondria: these are often thought of as the 'power houses' of cells because this is where energy is produced. The mitochondria break down sugar molecules in the presence of oxygen to produce energy in the form of ATP.
- Rough/smooth endoplasmic reticulum (ER): a series of interconnecting tubular tunnels, which are continuous with the outer membrane of the nucleus. The membrane structure of both types is identical but the rough ER has ribosomes attached to it as opposed to smooth ER, which does not. The rough ER is involved in protein synthesis, allowing proteins made on the ribosomes to

fold into their three-dimensional shape; the smooth ER is the site
of steroid production.

- Lysosomes: these are spherical bodies containing many digestive
  enzymes that are used to break down large molecules.
- Golgi apparatus: this is a stack of flattened sacs, associated with
  the ER. The Golgi apparatus modifies proteins and fats, e.g. the
  addition of sugar molecules to form glycoproteins.

It is important to remember that not all cell organelles have been
described within this text. (A more detailed description of cell
organelles can be found in Alberts et al., 1994.)

How does the cell develop and replicate?

Eukaryotic cells divide to produce two identical daughter cells each
containing exact copies of the DNA from the parent cell; in this way
multicellular organisms are able to replace damaged or worn-out
cells. These processes are called interphase and mitosis and together
they make up the cell cycle (Figure 4.2).

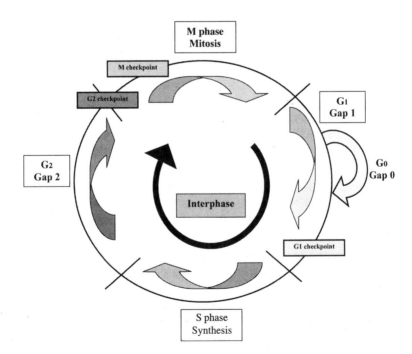

Figure 4.2 Overview of the five stages of normal mammalian cell development.
Within each stage there are checkpoints that are regulated by components within
the cycle.

To the naked eye interphase appears to be a period of rest for the cell, but in fact much activity is taking place. During this time RNA is constantly being synthesized, protein is produced and the cell is growing in size. Scientists have determined at a molecular level that the interphase can be divided into the following four steps.

Gap 0 (G0)

Cells may leave the cell cycle for a temporary resting period or more permanently if they have reached the end of their development, e.g. neurons. Cells in this phase are often termed quiescent. To enter back into the cycle, cells must be stimulated by growth factors, e.g. platelet-derived growth factor (PDGF).

Gap 1 (G1)

Cells increase in size, produce RNA and synthesize protein. There is an important cell cycle control mechanism (checkpoint) activated during this stage (see 'Tumour suppressor genes', p. 38) that cells must pass through in order to progress to S phase.

Synthesis phase (S phase)

DNA is replicated during this phase so that the two daughter cells produced after mitosis will contain a copy of the DNA from the parent cells.

Gap 2 (G2)

Cells continue to grow and produce new proteins. At the end of G2 another important checkpoint is activated (see 'Tumour suppressor genes').

Now the cell is ready to enter mitosis, this is further divided into the following stages.

Prophase

At the beginning of prophase the nuclear membrane breaks down and chromatin in the nucleus condenses into chromosomes (these can be viewed under a light microscope). Each chromosome consists of two genetically identical chromatids. Microtubules, which are responsible for cell shape, disassemble and the building blocks of these are used to form the mitotic spindle.

Prometaphase

There is now no longer a recognizable nucleus. Some mitotic spindle fibres elongate to specific areas on the chromosomes.

Metaphase

Tension is applied to the spindle fibres, which align all the chromosomes in one plane at the centre of the cell.

Anaphase

The chromosomes are pulled away from the central plane towards the cell poles.

Telophase

Chromosomes arrive at cell poles and decondense; the nuclear envelope re-forms around the clusters at each end of the cell, thereby forming new nuclei.

Cytokinesis

The cell is cleaved to form two daughter cells and microtubules re-form for the cell's entry into interphase.

These cells are said to be diploid because they contain two sets of homologous chromosomes. Another form of cell division to be aware of is meiosis, which occurs only in reproductive cells during the formation of gametes (sex cells). A cell dividing by meiosis duplicates its DNA as with cells undergoing mitosis, but splits into four new cells instead of two and contains only one copy of each chromosome. These cells are said to be haploid.

How is the cell cycle controlled?

Cancer can be described as the uncontrolled proliferation and growth of cells into other tissues. If we can understand the normal mechanisms in place for control of the cell cycle, we can begin to understand how these controls may malfunction and cause cancer to develop. Understanding the cell cycle and its controls also allows the development of specific and targeted therapies to treat the disease.

Cyclins and cyclin-dependent kinases

Many different proteins located within the cytoplasm control the cell cycle; two of the main types are cyclins (structural proteins) and cyclin-dependent kinases (CDKs). A cyclin joins with a CDK to form a complex (cyclin–CDK); however, if a problem with the cell cycle is detected, activation of the cyclin–CDK complex is not completed. If there are no problems activation is completed, which leads to the activation of a transcription factor by the removal of a transcription factor inhibitor. The transcription factor activates transcription of the genes required for the next stage of the cell cycle, including the cyclin and *CDK* genes. During the cell cycle, levels of cyclins within the cell will rise and fall but the levels of CDKs will remain fairly constant. Activation of CDKs is a central event in regulating the cell cycle and their activity is therefore regulated at many different levels.

Tumour suppressor genes

Tumour suppressor genes prevent excessive growth of a cell; the most well-known ones are *p53* and the retinoblastoma (*Rb*) gene.

Retinoblastoma gene

Rb is involved in the G1 checkpoint (see Figure 4.2) in the following way: it binds to a family of transcription factors known as the E2F family, thereby repressing their transcription of E2F-responsive genes such as thymidine kinase (TK) which are needed for DNA replication and cyclin E and A needed for cell cycle progression. *Rb* is activated when cyclin D forms a complex with CDK4/6 (cyclin D–CDK4/6, hence making it active); this in turn phosphorylates *Rb*, which allows E2F to be released (Figure 4.3).

The p53 gene

The p53 protein is essential for protecting us against cancer; more than half of human cancers have *p53* mutations and therefore no functioning *p53*. It works by sensing DNA damage and halting the cell cycle (see Figure 4.2). This is essential because, if DNA is damaged but still replicated in the S phase, it could eventually manifest in the form of a protein mutation; so, by halting the cell cycle at the G1 checkpoint, this mutation can be prevented. How does this process work? Again, it comes back to the involvement of CDKs. First, in response to a variety of stress signals, e.g. DNA damage, *p53* switches from an inactive to an active state. It then triggers transcription of the gene for p21, which is a CDK inhibitor; as active CDKs are needed to progress through the cell cycle, an inactive CDK will cause the cycle to halt.

The *p53* gene is also involved at the G2 checkpoint in cases, for example, where DNA has been synthesized incorrectly. At this checkpoint, *p53* binds to E2F (see above) and prevents it from triggering transcription of proto-oncogenes, e.g. *c-myc* and *c-fos*, which are required for mitosis (see Figure 4.3). Proto-oncogenes are important promoters of normal cell growth and division; however, if they become mutated, they are known as oncogenes and can have a detrimental effect. A single oncogene cannot cause cancer by itself but it

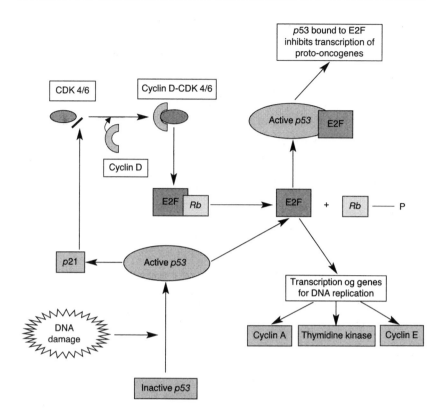

Figure 4.3 If no damage is detected at the G1 checkpoint, cyclic-dependent kinase CDK4/6 joins with cyclin D to form a cyclin–CDK complex. This phosphorylates Rb thereby releasing E2F from its complex and making it active. E2F promotes transcription of E2F-responsive genes and hence cell cycles progression. If there is no DNA damage, *p53* changes from its inactive state to its active state. This triggers transcription of the CDK inhibitor p21, which subsequently blocks the CDK, forming a complex with a cyclin.

can cause the cell cycle to lose its inhibitory controls, thereby increasing the rate of mitosis. When a cell loses control over mitosis, it can be the beginning of the pathway leading to the development of cancer.

Apoptosis

There are six main types of DNA-repair mechanisms operating in mammals; however, these are not always successful. The alternative pathway that can be activated by *p53* is apoptosis or programmed cell death. This process involves a series of specific cellular changes that result in the death of the cell and therefore any mutations within it.

Different types of cells

The human body is made up of three types of cell: somatic, germ and stem cells. Somatic cells make up most of the body; there are two copies of each chromosome so they are diploid. Germ cells give rise to gametes and are constant throughout their generations. Stem cells, on the other hand, have the ability to divide indefinitely and give rise to specialized cells, e.g. blood stem cells can give rise to red blood cells, platelets and white blood cells. Table 4.1 describes some of the different types of tissues within the body and cells of which they are composed; most tissues are made up of more than one type of cell.

Table 4.1 Cell and tissue types found within the body and their function

Tissue/cell type	Function
Epithelia*	
Absorptive	Numerous hair-like structures called microvilli project from their surface to increase the surface area for absorption
Secretory	Specialized cells that secrete substances on to the surface of the cell sheet. They are often collected together to form a gland that specializes in the secretion of a particular substance. Exocrine glands secrete their products, e.g. gastric juices, into ducts; endocrine glands secrete into the blood
Ciliated	Cilia on their free surface which beat in synchrony to move substances, e.g. mucus, over the epithelial sheet
Connective tissue	
Fibroblasts	Located in loose connective tissue and secrete the extracellular matrix which fills spaces between organs and tissues
Osteoblasts	Secrete the extracellular matrix in which crystals of calcium phosphate are later deposited to form bone
Adipose	Among the largest in the body and produce and store fat. A large lipid droplet within the cell squeezes the nucleus and cytoplasm
Nervous tissue	
Neurons	Specialized cells for communication, e.g. the brain and spinal cord comprise a network of neurons
Glial	Cells that support neurons
Schwann or oligodendrocytes	Wrap around the axon forming a multilayered membrane sheath. The axon is the structure that conducts electrical signals away from the neuron

Table 4.1 (contd)

Tissue/cell type	Function
Muscle tissue	
Skeletal	Large multinucleated cells that form muscle fibres. Skeletal muscle moves joints by its strong rapid contraction
Smooth	Composed of thin elongated cells containing one nucleus each. Found in the digestive tract, bladder, arteries and veins
Cardiac	An intermediate of the previous two types. Cardiac muscle produces the heart beat, cells are linked by electrically conducting junctions
Blood	
Erythrocytes (red blood cells)	Very small cells usually with no nucleus or internal membrane. Full of oxygen-binding protein haemoglobin
Lymphocytes (white blood cells)	These cells protect us against infections. They are further subdivided into lymphocytes, macrophages and neutrophils
Sensory	
Hair	Sensory cells which are some of the most highly specialized cells within the vertebrate body. Hair cells of the inner ear are primary detectors of sound
Rod	These are found in the retina of the eye and are specialized to respond to light

•Epithelial cells form cell sheets called epithelia; these line inner and outer surfaces of the body.

What happens when the cell undergoes malignant changes?

Over the years it has been suggested that the development of cancer is a multistep process, each step reflecting a genetic alteration that transforms a normal cell into a malignant cell. A review by Hanahan and Weinberg (2000) summarized these changes as six essential alterations to cell physiology which collectively dictate malignant growth. The alterations are as follows.

Self-sufficiency in growth signals

Normal cells require growth signals to proliferate. Many cancer cells acquire the ability to produce their own growth signals, i.e. they can synthesize growth factors, to which they also respond. The cells begin to operate as an independent entity as opposed to functioning as part of a larger organism. An example of this is the ability of glioblastomas to produce PDGF (Hermansson et al., 1988).

Insensitivity to inhibitory (antigrowth) signals

Cells monitor their external environment and decide whether or not to proliferate. Many anti-proliferative signals function via the Rb protein (see 'Tumour suppressor genes'); if this is disrupted, therefore, control of the cell cycle is lost and cells will proliferate. This is demonstrated in retinoblastoma cancer where deletion or mutation of the *Rb* gene causes tumour growth in one or both eyes in early childhood.

Evasion of apoptosis

Research over the past decade has determined that the apoptotic programme is present in nearly all cells of the body in a latent form. It seems that resistance towards it is a characteristic of most and perhaps all cancers. One way in which apoptosis might be avoided is the loss or mutation of *p53*, which acts as a proapoptotic regulator by sensing DNA damage.

Limitless replicative potential

Research involving cells in culture has suggested that normal cells can undergo only 60–70 replications, after which time they stop growing and die. Cancer cells have, however, acquired the capability to replicate endlessly, in many cases as a result of an enzyme known as telomerase. At the end of chromosomes are telomeres, which are composed of several thousand repeats of base-pairs. During each normal cell replication the telomeres shorten until they can no longer protect the chromosomal DNA, and subsequently the cell dies. However, if telomerase is upregulated, the telomeres will be maintained above a critical length, making the cells immortal.

Sustained angiogenesis

Angiogenesis is the formation of new blood vessels, which is an essential process if the cells in the tumour mass are to be supplied with oxygen and nutrients. It seems that tumours are able to shift the balance of angiogenesis inducers and inhibitors by altering gene expression and, for example, increasing expression of vascular endothelial growth factor (VEGF) (Hanahan and Folkman, 1996).

Tissue invasion and metastasis

Most cancer deaths are caused by metastasis of the primary tumour mass to other sites of the body. It begins with the rearrangement of the cell's cytoskeleton, which allows them to attach to other cells and move over or around them. Once they hit a blockage, e.g. the basal lamina, the cancer cells secrete enzymes to break it down. Included in these enzymes are matrix metalloproteins (MMPs), which act as 'molecular scissors' and cut through proteins that may hinder the passage of the cancer cells. Once through the basal lamina, the cells can move into the bloodstream and circulate throughout the body until they find a suitable site to settle on and regrow. A commonly observed alteration that leads to metastasis involves the cell-to-cell interaction molecule E-cadherin. Coupling of this molecule between cells results in transmission of antigrowth signals, thereby acting as a suppressor of invasion and metastasis. It appears that E-cadherin's function is lost in most epithelial cancers as a result of gene mutations.

How may a particular malignant condition present?

Different conditions may present themselves in various ways and the earlier the condition is recognized the better the chance of cure.

Colorectal cancer

Symptoms may include blood or mucus in the faeces, changes in bowel habits (diarrhoea/constipation or both), anything abnormal or that lasts for more than 2 weeks, the feeling of needing to go to the toilet even if the bowels have just been emptied, pain or discomfort in the abdominal area, a mass in the abdomen or extreme tiredness, which could be the result of anaemia. These symptoms may well be caused by other conditions, e.g. a common cause of bleeding is haemorrhoids. However, it is important that anyone experiencing these symptoms should see their doctor (Cancer Research UK website, 2002b).

Breast cancer

It is important that women know what is normal for them personally and that they are aware of the following signs: lumps or thickening in the breast or axillary area; changes in the skin in these areas, e.g. dimpling, redness or puckering; changes in the nipple, e.g. a change in the shape or an unusual discharge; changes around the nipple, e.g. an unusual rash or sore area; and changes to the shape and size of the breast and unusual pain or discomfort, although pain unaccompanied by any other symptoms is unlikely to be caused by cancer. These symptoms may be explained by other reasons but should still be reported to the doctor (Cancer Research UK website, 2002a).

Lung cancer

Symptoms for this disease may not be experienced in the early stages of development and, when symptoms do occur, they are usually the result of the cancer growing and causing pressure or pain, e.g. a persistent cough, wheezing and shortness of breath and blood in the phlegm; recurrent chest infections, chest, shoulder or back pain not related to coughing, a husky voice, unexplained weight loss or loss of appetite; and unsteady walking or occasional memory lapses and pathological fractures (Cancer Research UK website, 2002c).

Effects of cytotoxic chemotherapy

Cytotoxic drugs target dividing cells; this means that cytotoxics have both anti-cancer effects and the potential to harm normal tissue, in particular cells that are continuously renewed, e.g. the epithelial lining of the stomach or hair follicles. There are many drugs available to treat the many different types of cancer. In this text and Table 4.2 we concentrate on categories of chemotherapeutic agents that are cytotoxic, i.e. drugs that act against cancer by killing the cancer cells themselves. There are other types of drugs to be aware of that do not fall into the 'cytotoxic' category, e.g. Herceptin, a drug developed from substances found in the immune system, is more likely to be referred to as immunotherapy.

How chemotherapy affects different stages of the cell cycle

Alkylating agents

These drugs were the first non-hormonal drugs to be used to treat cancer effectively. They were developed after the observations that sulphur and nitrogen mustards used during World War I caused bone marrow suppression and lymphoid aplasia. Trials in patients with lymphoma demonstrated regression of tumours and this prompted the search for more effective but less toxic nitrogen mustards (Colvin, 2000). Cyclophosphamide is an alkylating agent used to treat many different cancers, including lymphoma, breast and lung cancer. It is a prodrug, which means that it must be activated before it becomes cytotoxic. Its mechanism of action is cell cycle phase

Table 4.2 Description of cytotoxic drugs within different classes, their mechanism of action and main tumours that they are used to treat

Drug class	Cell cycle specific	Mechanism of action	Examples of tumours treated
Alkylating agents			
Carmustine	X	Can cause cross-linking in nuclear macromolecules; some cell cycle specificity	Brain, lymphoma
Cyclophosphamide	X	Causes single-/double-strand breaks to DNA	Breast, endometrial, lung, lymphoma, ovarian cancer
Temozolomide	X	Methylation of DNA at the O^6 position on guanine	Astrocytoma, glioblastoma, brain metastases, melanoma
Treosulfan	X	Causes cross-linking of DNA	Ovarian, unknown primary cancer
Cytotoxic antibiotics			
Doxorubicin	X	Intercalates DNA/RNA, produces free radicals and inhibits topoisomerase II	Leukaemia, breast, lung, ovarian, sarcoma
Mitomycin C	X	Binds to DNA, causing cross-linking, and inhibition of DNA synthesis and function	Bladder, colorectal, gastric, skin cancer
Mitozantrone	X	Causes intra-/interstrand DNA cross-linking and binds to phosphate backbone of DNA, causing strand breaks	Breast cancer, leukaemia
Antimetabolites			
Methotrexate	✓	S-phase specific; inhibits synthesis of ribonucleosides	Breast, head and neck cancer, leukaemia

(contd)

Table 4.2 (contd)

Drug class	Cell cycle specific	Mechanism of action	Examples of tumours treated
5-Fluorouracil (5FU)	✓	S-phase specific; stops DNA synthesis by inhibiting thymidine production	Breast, colorectal, gastric cancer
Vinca alkaloids			
Vincristine	✓	M-phase specific with metaphase arrest; inhibits microtubule assembly	Hodgkin's and non-Hodgkin's lymphoma, leukaemia, lung cancer, rhabdomyosarcoma
Vindesine	✓	M-phase specific with metaphase arrest; inhibits microtubule assembly	Advanced breast cancer, malignant melanoma
Vinorelbine	✓	M-phase specific with metaphase arrest; inhibits microtubule assembly and is more selective than previous two drugs	Breast, lung cancer
Platinum compounds			
Carboplatin	✗	Causes intra-/interstrand DNA cross-linking	Ovarian cancer, lung cancer
Cisplatin	✗	Causes intra-/interstrand DNA cross-linking; possible cell cycle effects	Bladder, lung, ovarian, testicular cancer
Oxaliplatin	✗	Causes intra-/interstrand DNA cross-linking, possible synergy with 5FU and irinotecan	Colorectal cancer
Taxanes			
Paclitaxel	✓	Promotes microtubule assembly and inhibits de-assembly thereby inhibiting cell replication	Breast, melanoma, ovarian cancer

Docetaxel	✓	G2/M-phase specific; promotes microtubule assembly and inhibits de-assembly thereby inhibiting cell replication	Breast, lung cancer
Topoisomerase inhibitors			
Irinotecan	✓	S-phase specific; inhibits topoisomerase I	Colorectal cancer
Topotecan	✓	S-phase specific; inhibits topoisomerase I	Ovarian cancer
Miscellaneous			
Etoposide	✓	Late S-phase and G2 specific; inhibits topoisomerase II	Lung, testicular cancer

non-specific, i.e. it does not act at a specific point within the cell cycle; instead it binds to DNA causing single- or double-strand breaks, thereby preventing cell division.

Cytotoxic antibiotics

Doxorubicin is an anthracycline antibiotic produced by the fungus *Streptomyces peucetius*. Similar to previous agents it is cell cycle phase non-specific and acts instead by intercalating between DNA and RNA. It has been shown to produce toxic oxygen free radicals which cause single- and double-strand breaks to DNA, and also to inhibit topoisomerase II, an enzyme that is critical to DNA function.

Antimetabolites

Methotrexate is an analogue of folic acid that has been used clinically since 1948 to treat cancers including breast, colorectal and gastric. It is cell cycle specific for the S phase, hence it inhibits DNA synthesis. It functions by competing for folate-binding sites on an enzyme known as dihydrofolate reductase, which normally converts dihydrofolate to tetrahydrofolate. The latter is needed by the cell as a prerequisite to synthesizing thymidylate and purine precursors, essential components of DNA synthesis.

Vinca alkaloids

This class of drug is used to treat acute leukaemias, lymphomas and some solid tumours such as breast and lung cancer. The mechanism of action is cell cycle specific and functions by blocking mitosis with metaphase arrest. Specifically, the drug binds to tubulin, a substructure of the microtubular spindle apparatus, thereby interrupting mitosis and causing cell death.

Platinum compounds

Cisplatin was first synthesized in 1845 but its cytotoxic properties were not described until 1965; it was entered into clinical trials in 1971. Once cisplatin is inside the cell, highly reactive charged platinum complexes are formed which cause intrastrand, interstrand and protein cross-linking of DNA. It was originally thought that cisplatin was cell cycle phase non-specific, but recent studies have shown complex and variable effects on the cell cycle.

Taxanes

Paclitaxel is an extract from the bark of the Pacific yew, *Taxus brevifolia*. It is a spindle inhibitor but, unlike vinca alkaloids that inhibit microtubule assembly, paclitaxel actually promotes assembly and stabilizes them against disassembly, thereby inhibiting cell replication.

Topoisomerase I inhibitors

Irinotecan is licensed to treat metastatic colorectal cancer in combination with the anti-metabolite 5-fluorouracil (5FU). Irinotecan is cell cycle specific for the S phase and inhibits the action of topoisomerase I, an enzyme that produces reversible single-strand breaks in DNA during DNA replication to allow relief of tension within the molecule. Irinotecan binds to the enzyme–DNA complex and prevents the DNA from rejoining; this causes double-strand breakage and cell death.

Last is etoposide, an agent that does not fit into any of the previously mentioned classes. It causes single-strand breaks in DNA and also is cell cycle specific for late S phase and G2. It causes DNA damage through inhibition of topoisomerase II and activates reactions that produce molecules which bind directly to DNA.

Further sources

American Heritage Dictionary of the English Language (2000) Retrieved March 3, 2003, from www.bartleby.com/61/81/N0188100.html

British National Formulary (2002) Malignant disease and immunosuppression.

Drug Index (Professional) (2001) Retrieved February 2003, from www.bccancer.bc.ca/HPI/DrugDatabase/DrugIndexALPro/default.htm

Colorectal (bowel) cancer (2002) Retrieved March 3, 2003, from Cancer Research UK web site: www.cancerresearchuk.org

Breast cancer (2002) Retrieved March 3, 2003, from Cancer Research UK web site: www.cancerresearchuk.org

Lung cancer (2002) Retrieved March 3, 2003, from Cancer Research UK web site: www.cancerresearchuk.org

CHAPTER 5
What are DNA and RNA?

SCOTT C. EDMUNDS

It is now common knowledge that DNA (deoxyribonucleic acid) is the carrier of genetic information in all living cells. It has, however, been a long, slow process to explain how this relatively simple-structured molecule carries all of the genetic information and enables the existence of all of the richly varied life on our planet. The DNA molecule stores information coding for all the instructions needed to make a living organism. It does this in a similar way to how a computer program uses instructions that are encoded in a digital computer code. But where computer memory uses a binary system of ones and zeroes (e.g. 1101 10111010010110), the genetic code uses repeating subunits of the DNA molecule (e.g. TAG GAT TAC CAT). This molecule has to be able to do many complicated tasks such as being able to replicate perfectly. It also needs to be able to translate the message into an intermediate message molecule (now known to be RNA) that can travel to the protein-producing machinery of the cell, and then make all of the tens of thousands of different proteins that make up an organism (Figure 5.1).

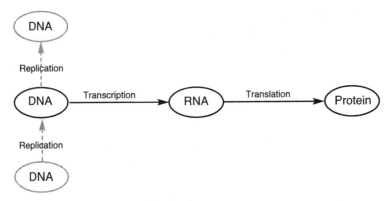

Figure 5.1 DNA makes RNA makes protein – the fundamental dogma of molecular biology.

Background

Looking at the resemblances between parent and child it is obvious that physical traits are inherited. The ancient Greeks were the first to formulate a scientific theory for how this could work – the theory of 'pangenesis', where representative particles from all over the body pass as hereditary material through the semen. This theory pretty much held sway until the eighteenth and nineteenth centuries. It was not until the 1860s that Gregor Mendel, a Czech Monk who did breeding experiments with common garden peas, first reported the basic laws of genetic inheritance. From these experiments Mendel hypothesized that phenotypical (physical) traits are the result of the interaction of 'discrete particles' (now called genes) provided by both parents and passed to their offspring.

Mendel's theories were almost universally ignored by his contemporaries during his lifetime, but were rediscovered in 1900, many years after his death. The discovery of chromosomes at around this time – and their similarity in behaviour to Mendel's 'discrete particles' – led to Walter Sutton's 'chromosomal theory of inheritance' in 1903. Although scientists were convinced that the hereditary material resided in these chromosomes, it was puzzling as to what substance carried this information. From chemical analysis it was discovered that the chromosomes were made of both DNA and protein. Initially it was not thought that DNA could carry the genetic code; it seemed too simple a molecule – linear and made up of monotonous repeating sequences of four subunits. Proteins are far more complicated molecules, with up to 20 different subunits, and complicated three-dimensional branched and globular structures.

It was not until the 1940s and 1950s that scientists started to accept evidence that DNA was the carrier of genetic information. In 1944 Avery discovered that bacteria called pneumococci could be transformed from an innocuous to a virulent form by the addition of purified DNA extract from other virulent bacteria. It took several years for these findings to become accepted, but from this point onwards the challenge was to determine the structure of DNA, and how the molecule worked as the carrier of genetic information (Avery et al., 1944).

Determining the structure of DNA

DNA is a long chain of nucleotides consisting of three parts:

- Deoxyribose, a pentose (five-carbon) sugar
- Phosphoric acid

- One of four organic (nitrogenous) bases. These organic bases were either the purines adenine (A) and guanine (G) or the pyrimidines cytosine (C) and thymine (T).

How these four repeating subunits come together to form the genetic code now had to be explained. A major clue was discovered by Erwin Chargaff, who noted that, despite the seemingly large variation in the composition of these four bases from organism to organism, DNA always had an equal number of adenine and thymine residues (A = T) and of guanine and cytosine bases (G = C). This relationship is now known as 'Chargaff's rule'. The other crucial piece of evidence came from X-ray diffraction photography experiments on the DNA molecule, carried out by Maurice Wilkins and Rosalind Franklin at King's College in London, showing that this must be a helical molecule.

Using these two findings, two young scientists at Cambridge University, James Watson and Francis Crick, finally determined the structure of DNA – giving rise to the so-called 'Watson–Crick' model. This discovery and its publication in the journal *Nature* in 1953 was said by many to mark the birth of molecular biology (Watson and Crick, 1953). Crick, Watson and Wilkins won the Nobel Prize for chemistry in 1964 (tragically by this time Rosalind Franklin had died), and the way was now clear for tremendous strides in our understanding of DNA – arguably the central molecule of life. In addition to providing the structure of this molecule, the Watson–Crick model also suggests the molecular mechanism for heredity.

The primary structure of DNA

Individual nucleotides form a polynucleotide linear polymer where each mononucleotide monomer unit is linked by chemical bonds known as phosphodiester bridges. These bonds link the 3'-carbon in the ribose of one deoxynucleotide to the 5'-carbon in the ribose of the adjacent deoxynucleotide (for an overview, see Voet and Voet, 1995) (Figure 5.2).

The genome of all living cells is composed of double-stranded DNA containing two anti-parallel polynucleotide chains. This is because the organic bases project into the centre of the molecule (with the phosphate and ribose groups acting as a backbone on the outside) and form base-pairs joined by non-covalent hydrogen bonds. Adenine links to thymine only via two hydrogen bonds, and guanidine links to cytosine via three hydrogen bonds. This makes two anti-parallel strands with their 5' to 3' directions being in opposite directions to each other. This

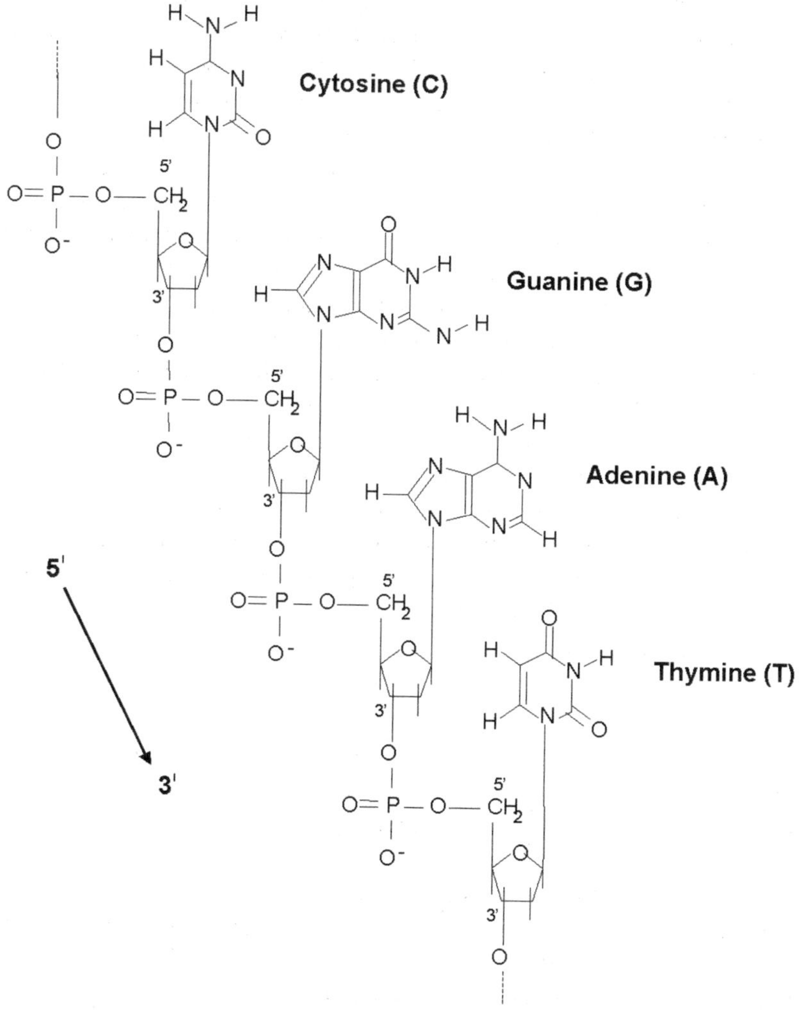

Figure 5.2 The structure of the DNA molecule.

specificity of base-pairing thus allows precise duplication of DNA, while holding the two strands tightly together. The geometry of these Watson–Crick base-pairs makes these two DNA strands wrap around together, forming a double helix. In double-stranded DNA there is one turn of the helix every 3.4 nm.

Some facts

The bacterium *Escherichia coli* has a single circular DNA molecule of 4.6 million base-pairs, making the total length of this single DNA molecule around 1.4 mm. In humans there are around 3 billion letters in the DNA code. In a single diploid cell, if fully extended, the DNA would have a length of almost 2 metres. If all the DNA of the roughly 100 trillion cells in the human body were unwrapped and placed end to end, it would reach the moon 6000 times!

Fortunately, DNA in the human cell is not unwound, because it needs to be contained within a nucleus only 10 μm in diameter. DNA is packaged by wrapping the DNA up with proteins called histones. The DNA molecule wraps around several types of histone proteins, collected up into a structure known as a nucleosome. These nucleosomes, with DNA wrapped around, fold up further, coiling all of this DNA and protein and forming the chromosomes. How tightly folded this DNA is varies according to what the DNA is encoding, and what process the DNA is undergoing at the time.

The genetic information needs to be able to carry out three functions. A gene needs to replicate itself, making a perfect copy every time the cell divides, a process known as replication. This gene must be able to translate the genetic message to make a protein, known as transcription. Finally, from this message the protein has to be manufactured from individual amino acid units, a process known as translation (Williams et al., 1995).

Replication

The specific Watson–Crick base-pairing and double helical structure of the DNA molecule has made it quite easy to deduce the copying mechanism for the genetic material. The two parent strands of the double helix are unwound, with each strand acting as a template for the synthesis of a complementary daughter strand. Free nucleotides floating in the nucleoplasm have a free triphosphate group on the 5'-carbon atom of the sugar, and this bonds with a hydroxyl group on the template. This means that the chain can grow only in a 5' to 3' direction. This process is catalysed by the enzyme DNA polymerase. As the DNA chains can grow only in a 5'-to-3' direction, one of the strands is replicated in a series of short discontinuous pieces as the parental helix unwinds. These short fragments are subsequently joined up by another enzyme, known as DNA ligase. The parental duplex is thus replicated to form two daughter duplexes, each consisting of one parental strand and one newly synthesized daughter strand (Figure 5.3).

Transcription

The genetic information held in the DNA has to direct the production of all of the proteins that build up in a cell and then in a whole organism. As proteins are produced in the cytoplasm, and the DNA is

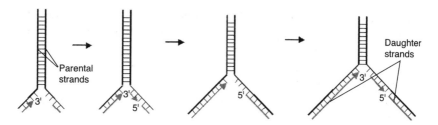

Figure 5.3 DNA replication.

held in the nucleus, an intermediary 'transcript' molecule has to pass this information to the protein-making machinery. This intermediary molecule is another nucleic acid very similar to DNA, known as ribonucleic acid or RNA. RNA differs in structure from DNA in that its pentose sugar is a ribose rather than deoxyribose, and the organic base thymine is replaced by a different pyrimidine called uracil. Uracil (U) acts as the complementary base to adenine, and all of the bases in RNA can bind and form a complementary strand to a DNA template. This allows a RNA copy of the genetic message to be produced in a fundamentally similar way to DNA replication, except that only one of the DNA strands is ever copied. This makes RNA a single-stranded molecule.

There are three major classes of RNA: messenger RNA (mRNA), ribosomal RNA (rRNA) and transfer RNA (tRNA). As its name suggests, mRNA is the carrier of the genetic message; the other RNAs (tRNA and rRNA) are structural RNAs that are part of the protein-making machinery. In a typical cell, thousands of different mRNAs can be produced and transported around the cell, each one transcribed from different genes and each different transcript coding for a different protein.

There are 20 amino acids and the four nucleotides that make up the genetic code need to be able to encode the instructions for proteins containing any number of these 20 units, along with at least one code giving instructions for when the protein-making machinery should start or stop. To code for this number of amino acids and start/stop instructions, a language based on nucleotide triplets is used and is normally represented as groups of three letters, e.g. TAG, CGE, AGC, etc. This gives a potential number of 64 possible triplets that can be coded for ($4^3 = 64$). Thus, the mRNA sequence is read as a number of triplets, or 'codons', each codon specifying the insertion of a specific amino acid into the growing protein chain. Initiation of translation begins at an initiation codon, AUG, which is also the code for the amino acid methionine. Termination of protein synthesis is coded by one of three different termination codons: UAA, UAG or UGA. As there are 64 possible codons in the genetic code and only 20 different amino acids are used, the code is said to be degenerate, most amino acids being coded by more than one codon. This means that some amino acids, e.g. alanine, can be encoded by four codons (GCU, GCC, GCA and GCC), whereas others, e.g. tryptophan, are encoded by only one (UGG) (Strachan and Read, 1999) (Table 5.1).

Table 5.1 The genetic code

First letter	Second letter				Third letter
	U	C	A	G	
U	UUU (Phe)	UCU (Ser)	UAU (Tyr)	UGU (Cys)	U
	UUC (Phe)	UCC (Ser)	UAC (Tyr)	UGC (Cys)	C
	UUA (Leu)	UCA (Ser)	UAA (Stop)	UGA (Stop)	A
	UUG (Leu)	UCG (Ser)	UAG (Stop)	UGG (Trp)	G
C	CUU (Leu)	CCU (Pro)	CAU (His)	CGU (Arg)	U
	CUC (Leu)	CCC (pro)	CAC (His)	CGC (Arg)	C
	CUA (Leu)	CCA (Pro)	CAA (Gln)	CGA (Arg)	A
	CUG (Leu)	CCG (Pro)	CAG (Gln)	CGG (Arg)	G
A	AUU (Ile)	ACU (Thr)	AAU (Asn)	AGU (Ser)	U
	AUC (Ile)	ACC (Thr)	AAC (Asn)	AGC (Ser)	C
	AUA (Ile)	ACA (Thr)	AAA (Lys)	AGA (Arg)	A
	AUG (Met)	ACG (Thr)	AAG (Lys)	AGG (Arg)	G
G	GUU (Val)	GCU (Ala)	GAU (Asp)	GGU (Gly)	U
	GUC (Val)	GCC (Ala)	GAC (Asp)	GGC (Gly)	C
	GUA (Val)	GCA (Ala)	GAA (Glu)	GGA (Gly)	A
	GUG (Val)	GCG (Ala)	GAG (Glu)	GGG (Gly)	G

The mRNA of eukaryotic organisms is modified in several ways before it can be translated. The mRNA molecule is capped at both ends, possibly to prevent premature degradation and possibly to help guide the molecule to the protein-making machinery. A modified nucleotide base, a methylated guanine residue, caps the 5′ end. The 3′ end is capped by 100–200 adenine residues, and is known as the poly-A tail. Most genes of higher organisms are interrupted by segments of non-coding DNA. These genes are made up of patches of coding (exons) interspersed with non-coding sequence (introns). These introns are removed from the mRNA or spliced before the mRNA leaves the nucleus. This mechanism of rearranging introns and exons gives the organism flexibility in mixing and matching different functional parts of genes to create different splice forms with different functions.

Translation

Translation is mRNA-directed biosynthesis of protein. The protein-making machinery produces the specific protein (polypeptide) by a cytoplasmic organelle known as the ribosome. The ribosome is part protein and part structural RNA, known as rRNA. When mRNA binds to the ribosome translation can start; each amino acid is carried to the site of protein synthesis by an intermediary molecule known as tRNA. There is a specific tRNA for each amino acid, each one binding to the mRNA triplet that encodes that amino acid. This binding is via an anticodon loop on the tRNA molecule which contains three nucleotides that base-pair to each mRNA codon. The ribosome provides a site for this binding to occur, starting first with the AUG initiation codon. The ribosome moves along the mRNA molecule in a 5′ to 3′ direction; each amino acid is brought by a tRNA molecule and then covalently bonded by enzymes to form a peptide (protein) chain. The ribosome falls off the mRNA chain when it reaches the termination codon, by which time it has produced a complete protein chain (Lewin, 1994).

The completed polypeptide chain contains signals that direct post-translational processing and transport to different cellular/extra-cellular compartments. More than one ribosome can bind to an mRNA molecule at any one time, and the number of ribosomes bound can determine the rate of translation (Figure 5.4).

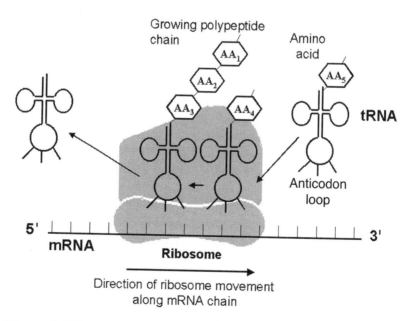

Figure 5.4 The translation of mRNA into protein.

Conclusion

The synthesis of all the body's proteins using the genetic code as a template has to be a very precise process. Protein after protein has to be produced in exactly the same way so that the function is not altered. The genetic code must not alter generation after generation of cell division in every single cell, out of the trillions that make up the human body. The specificity of the base pairing of the two anti-parallel strands is what allows precise duplication of this code. Various enzymes also proofread the DNA to make sure that any wrongly incorporated bases are removed. Despite this, errors in DNA replication do occur. If mutations occur inside transcribed parts of the genome, problems may arise. Mutations in the special promoter regions at the beginning of genes can mean that the protein may not be produced at all. Entire genes may be deleted, and mutations inside the exons of genes may produce mutant proteins that may have altered and disrupted function. These altered or missing proteins are implicated in many disorders and diseases, including cancer.

Chapter 6

Genetics and cancer

Scott C. Edmunds

What are genes?

As mentioned in Chapter 5, DNA is a molecule that contains the genetic code, encoding all the proteins that make up an organism. The human genome, the total amount of genetic material of which a human cell is composed, is made up of roughly 30 000–40 000 genes, single coding units of DNA that encode for each of the proteins produced by a human. If the genetic code of any gene is altered in any way (e.g. by a mutation) there can be potentially serious consequences for gene expression. This is particularly the case in genes that affect the health and life of the organism involved directly. If the structure or expression levels are abnormally altered in any of the countless proteins that are involved in the cellular processes essential for life, the consequences can be potentially life-threatening illnesses. This includes disorders such as cancer (Lewin, 2000).

Mutations

As most of the human genome is non-coding DNA sequence, so-called 'junk DNA', most genetic changes are usually harmless. Only about 3% of the human genome accounts for the coding sequence, and genes are split into coding and non-coding regions, known as introns (non-coding) and exons (coding), which are spliced together during transcription; therefore only mutations in exonic regions will affect the amino acid composition of a protein. Upstream (the 5' end) of the coding regions of any gene lie non-coding regions, essential for gene expression, known as promoter and enhancer elements. These give instructions for where the gene expression machinery should start transcription of the mRNA message, and what levels of transcript should be produced. Any alterations to genetic coding of these regions can potentially affect the expression of a gene. Finally, any alterations to regions around the splice sites of introns and exons, known as intron–exon junctions, can affect the splicing and exonic structure of a gene.

The nature of the genetic alteration can affect the severity of the consequence for the expression of the gene. Less severe mutations can involve single base substitutions, and some of these mutations are so-called 'silent mutations', which have no effect on the amino acid composition. More serious alterations to the gene are substitutions or deletions, with one or more nucleotides inserted or deleted. Larger-scale chromosomal abnormalities can also arise, where regions of the chromosome are gained or lost, or entire parts of the chromosome are broken and rejoined to other chromosomes. Mutations in DNA can be produced by errors in DNA replication and repair. The enzymes that control DNA replication are very efficient and there are many proofreading and repair mechanisms that can prevent dangerous mutations occurring. As a result of the sheer size of the human genome (3 billion base-pairs), the number of cells in the body and the number of times a cell will divide throughout a human's lifetime, it is no surprise that errors do sometimes occur. Mutations can also be induced by external factors such as mutagenic chemicals and radiation. Mutations either occur in the germ cells (sperm and eggs), which can be passed on from generation to generation, or in single cells, known as a somatic changes, which are not passed on.

Single base substitutions

Individual base substitutions are among the most common mutations and either they can be silent mutations or they can alter the sequence of the gene product transcribed. As each amino acid is specified by a single codon consisting of three bases, if a single base is substituted the altered sequence may code for a different codon. As a result of degeneracy of the code, several codons may code for the same amino acid, e.g. as there are two different codons that code for lysine, if the final base-pair of the codon was converted from an A to a G (i.e. AAA to AAG) this would be a silent mutation because both codons encode for the same amino acid. There are many other examples of this, because most amino acids are encoded by more than one codon.

It is common, however, for a single base substitution to alter the coding sequence. If the base-pair change results in a codon that codes for a different amino acid, this is known as a missense mutation. An example of this is if the first base of a codon encoding lysine were to be changed from an A to a G (i.e. AAA/AAG to GAA/GAG);

then the amino acid encoded would change to a glutamine. If the amino acid substituted in the protein is chemically very similar – with a similar charge or side chain – the change to the protein may not be that significant. If a radically different amino acid is substituted, especially in an important region of the protein molecule, the change can be quite serious. The type of single base substitution that makes the most significant change to a protein's structure is a nonsense mutation. Such a mutation produces an early stop codon, prematurely terminating the translation and leading to a potentially shortened protein. An example of this would be if the last base of a tyrosine codon was mutated from C or U to a G or A (i.e. UAC/UAU to UAA/UAG), producing a stop codon in this part of the message. How much of the protein is actually produced would depend on how near to the start of the transcript this mutation was.

Insertions and deletions

Nucleotides inserted into or deleted from coding regions of DNA can have very serious consequences for a gene, whether it is a single base that is lost or gained or larger sections of DNA transposed from another locus. As each specific codon consists of a triplet of nucleotides, the addition of a single nucleotide will lead to a frameshift effect, with each subsequent codon being read wrongly. This shift in the translational reading frame will also often lead to the introduction of a premature termination codon, causing a similar effect to a nonsense mutation. Larger insertions or deletions will add or remove large portions of coding sequence as well as potentially causing a frameshift, unless the number of nucleotides gained or lost is a multiple of three, in which case the reading frame is not altered (Lewin, 2000) (Figure 6.1).

Genetic disease

Germline (germ cells) mutations do accumulate over the generations and can have either a neutral or a harmful (pathogenic) effect on an organism. Mutations that are disadvantageous to an organism are slowly removed from the general population by natural selection, but this can take many, many generations. These harmful mutations can give rise to various diseases with a genetic basis: so-called genetic diseases. Over the past decade or so more and more diseases have been linked to genetic alterations. Monogenic disorders, caused by a mutation in a single gene, have been the simplest to understand and identify. Genes such as that for dystrophin, linked to Duchenne muscular dystrophy, or *CFTR*, linked to cystic fibrosis, have been

Normal sequence

mRNA   AGA CCA AAG UAC AUU AGG

Protein   Arg - Pro - Lys - Tyr - Ile - Arg

Missense mutation

A to G substitution

↓

mRNA   AGA CCA GAG UAC AUU AGG ...

Protein   Arg - Pro - Glu - Tyr - Ile - Arg - ...

Nonsense mutation

A to G substitution

↓

mRNA   AGA CCA AAG UAG AUU AGG ...

Protein   Arg - Pro - Lys - STOP

                    Termination

1bp Insertion

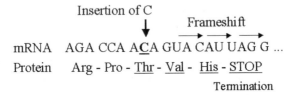

Insertion of C
                          Frameshift
↓   → → →
mRNA   AGA CCA ACA GUA CAU UAG G ...

Protein   Arg - Pro - Thr - Val - His - STOP

                        Termination

Figure 6.1 Some types of mutations.

found to be altered in patients with these diseases (Strachan and Read, 1999). Mutations in these essential genes alter their function, and patients with mutations in both chromosomal copies of these genes are unable to produce fully functional protein. These are recessive genetic disorders, and those people with only a single mutant allele are not affected. Some genetic disorders are dominant, with a mutant form of the protein having such a harmful (often toxic) effect on the patient that only a mutant single copy of the gene is needed to affect the patient. An example of this is the *HD* gene that plays a role in Huntington's disease (Gusella and MacDonald, 1993).

    Much more complicated are polygenic disorders, diseases that are significantly affected by the combinations of many disease susceptibility genes (along with environmental contributions) acting together. Diseases such as diabetes, and some forms of heart disease, are thought to act in a manner similar to this. Harmful genes act in an additive manner, and the effect of several of these disease-associated genes acting together will increase the susceptibility of an individual to that disease.

Cancer as a genetic disease

It is known that cancer is linked to harmful genetic alterations of cells and many genes have been linked to various forms of cancer, but the genetics of cancer is very complicated and less well understood than classic genetics. No single cancer-causing gene has ever been discovered that is mutated in all cancers, and even in specific tumour types there can be several possible genetic mechanisms and genes involved in the formation of the tumour. In some families an inherited disposition has been shown to play a role in cancer formation, but these familial cancers make up only a small proportion of cancer cases.

Cancer is a collection of disorders sharing the common feature of uncontrolled cell growth, leading to the formation of a mass of cells known as a 'neoplasm' or 'tumour'. Malignant neoplasms have the ability to invade adjacent tissues and often metastasize to more distant parts of the body, a process that is the cause of 90% of cancer deaths (Sporn, 1996). There are more than 200 types of cancer, and each is classified according to the tissue type in which they arise.

Cancers are almost always derived from a single ancestral somatic cell. The cells in an emerging neoplasm accumulate a series of genetic changes that lead to changes in gene activity and phenotype (Ponder, 2001). From studies on the incidence of cancer, it is thought that up to six or seven events are needed to turn a normal cell into a fully fledged invasive carcinoma. This is initially very confusing, because the probability of a single cell undergoing six independent mutations is virtually nil. There are mechanisms that can explain how this process can happen. These altered cells are subject to selection, and eventually a cell population evolves that can escape the controls of proliferation and territory. Initially mutations increase proliferation (growth), and this gives an increased target population of cells for the next mutation. At the same time some mutations will alter the stability of the whole genome, at either the DNA or chromosome level, and increase the overall mutation rate. This is a multi-step process, which explains why tumours always develop in stages, from benign growths to malignant tumour cells, at each step developing new mutations (Kinzler and Vogelstein, 1996) (Figure 6.2).

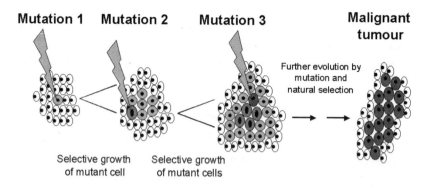

Figure 6.2 The multistage evolution of a cancer, with successive mutations giving cells a growth advantage; expanded populations of cells thus present a larger target for the next mutation. Cells are shaded progressively darker after each mutation.

Cancer-causing mutations generally affect genes that regulate cellular growth (the cell cycle) or death (apoptosis). It is thought that this process involves up to six essential alterations in cell physiology, including: self-sufficiency in the production of positive growth signals; disregard of inhibitory growth signals; an acquired capability for sustained growth (immortality of the cell); angiogenesis (blood vessel development); and finally metastasis (invasion and spread). Each of these changes represents the breaching of one of the body's anti-cancer mechanisms. These are predominantly somatic events, although in many of the inherited cancer syndromes one of these events may be inherited. Mutagenic environmental factors such as diet, radiation and exposure to carcinogenic compounds (e.g. cigarette smoke) can also affect the probability of these mutational events (Jorde et al., 2000).

The regulatory components that give the signals for cellular growth or inhibition of growth are usually external growth factors that act via complex signalling pathways affecting cellular growth (the cell cycle). It is various members of these pathways, and cell-cycle components, that are inactivated or down- or upregulated in many of the tumorigenic alterations to cell physiology. Growth signals include various cellular growth factors such as platelet-derived growth factor (PDGF) and transforming growth factor (TGF) α. These growth factors have signalling pathways that are also altered by many cancers to allow self-sufficiency in growth. Anti-growth signals can include growth factors such as TGFβ, and these need to be inactivated to allow cancer progression. These growth-inhibitory signals are also received by receptor molecules of the cell surface and coupled to other complicated networks of signalling pathways. Many of these signals are associated with the cell cycle, and can force cells out of the active proliferative cycle into a dormant state, where they remain until signalled at some future point. There are other complicated pathways governing apoptosis, senescence and angiogenesis which all have to be overcome in the development of a cancer (Hanahan and Weinberg, 2000). Once the cell has become hyperproliferative and cancerous, metastasis is a further multistep process, where the tumour cells have to detach from the primary tumour site and then reattach (via specific adhesion molecules) to the vascular tissues or other tissue sites to be invaded. Extracellular matrix proteins have to be degraded by enzymes released from the tumour or the surrounding cells.

Cancer genes can be divided into three main groups, according to whether they activate cellular proliferation (oncogenes), inhibit proliferation (tumour suppressors) or participate in DNA repair.

Oncogenes

Oncogenes were the first cancer-causing genes to be identified; they activate cellular proliferation, leading to unregulated cell growth and differentiation (Ponder, 2001). Most oncogenes are derived from a non-mutant version of the gene known as proto-oncogenes, which are usually involved in normal cellular growth. When a mutation occurs in a proto-oncogene, it can then become transformed to form an oncogene. Oncogenes can also be introduced from several types of DNA and RNA (retrovirus) viruses, which can integrate mutant oncogenes into the genome of a host. Oncogenes are usually dominant and activated by 'gain-of-function mutations'. Germline mutations in oncogenes are very uncommon, so this is predominantly a somatic event. Examples of oncogenes include *ras*, *myc*, *abl*, *fos* and *jun*. The gene *ras* is known to be mutated in up to 15% of all cancers.

Tumour suppressor genes

Tumour suppressor genes are 'anti-oncogenes', inhibiting cellular proliferation; they are usually inactivated by 'loss-of-function' mutations in cancer development. The first evidence for these loss-of-function genetic changes was from studies in the rare childhood eye cancer retinoblastoma. From studying sporadic and familial retinoblastoma, in 1971 Knudson formulated his two-hit model of carcinogenesis. In the familial form of the cancer, an affected parent has a 50% chance of passing the condition to an offspring and this is usually bilateral (in both eyes), whereas in the sporadic form there is no additional risk of inheritance and it is usually in one eye only.

Knudson hypothesized that this must be a two-hit event, with two rate-limiting steps for tumour formation.

In the inherited form, this is now known to result in predisposition to tumour formation because of germline mutations in one of our two copies of the tumour suppressor gene (Macleod, 2000). Somatic mutation of the second copy of the gene during the individual's lifetime results in tumour progression and formation. The second hit can be either by point mutation, or larger areas of chromosomal loss (allelic loss), or by other methods of silencing the gene. In the sporadic form two separate sporadic 'hits' are needed in the same cell for it to develop into a tumour clone. The minuscule chance of this rare event happening in both eyes is why formation of sporadic bilateral cancer is an incredibly unlikely event (Figure 6.3). The gene involved, *RB1*, which encodes the cell cycle regulatory protein pRb, has now been discovered on chromosome 13q14. Other important tumour suppressor genes include *p53*, *p16*, *BRCA-1*, *BRCA-2* and *PTEN* (Jorde et al., 2000). The *p53* gene *TP53* is known to be the most mutated gene involved in human cancer, with key roles in cell cycle control, apoptosis, angiogenesis and genetic

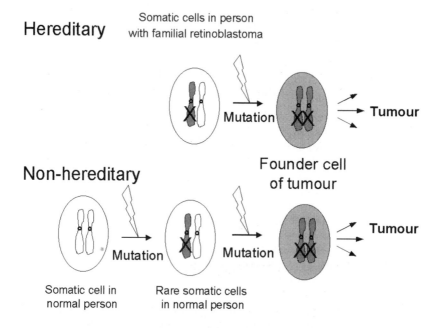

Figure 6.3 Knudson's two-hit hypothesis: tumour formation in both hereditary and non-hereditary retinoblastoma. A 'one-hit' clone is a precursor to the tumour in non-hereditary retinoblastomas, whereas all cells are one-hit clones in hereditary retinoblastoma.

stability. As it has such a central role in so many cancer-controlling pathways and activities, this may explain why this is probably the single most important tumour suppressor gene, and why it does not function correctly in most human cancers. In around half of these tumours *p53* is inactivated by mutations in *TP53*.

DNA-repair genes

The final class of genes implicated in carcinogenesis is involved in the various DNA-repair mechanisms that allow accurate DNA replication. In some inherited disorders and familial cancer syndromes, defects in these repair mechanisms lead to genomic instability. Genomic instability leads to chromosomal abnormalities such as breaks, abnormal chromosome numbers and widespread mutations; these somatic changes often affect genes that are important in proliferation and carcinogenesis (Jorde et al., 2000). Several colorectal and gastric cancer syndromes are known to have defects in the replication of short tandem repeat sequences (microsatellite sequences), known as microsatellite instability. This replication error defect is caused by mutations in the mismatch repair genes *MLH1* and *MSH2*, leading to a cascade of secondary mutations in oncogenes and tumour suppressor genes, which gives rise to cancer (Loeb, 1994). These replication error defects are also seen in some cases of sporadic cancer.

Chromosomal instability is seen in a larger number of cancers, where there are abnormal numbers of chromosomes, or smaller regions of chromosomal loss/gain or rearrangement. This process may be related to a mitotic checkpoint involving the *hBUB1* gene (Cahill et al., 1998), and can also be stimulated by processes that affect the three-dimensional structure of the DNA molecule such as ultraviolet radiation and chemical mutagens (Breivik and Gaudernack, 1999), and stimulate abnormal DNA repair. Chromosomal abnormalities increase during the progression of a cancer and lead to further alterations in cell physiology.

Methylation in tumorigenesis

Evidence has been accumulating that suggests that the methylation of cytosine bases has an important role in gene silencing (Antequera et al., 1990). This 'epigenetic' mechanism of gene inactivation has now been discovered to play a greater and greater role in carcinogenesis (Baylin and Herman, 2000). In the mammalian genome methylation occurs only at cytosines that are located 5′ to guanosine bases, known as the CpG dinucleotide (Bird, 1992). These CpG dinucleotides have been successively depleted in the human genome over its evolution, a phenomenon referred to as GC suppression. The remaining CpGs have a high frequency of methylation. This is thought to facilitate the repression of 'parasitic' repeated regions of the genome, such as retroviral genomic elements and self-replicating DNA junk regions known as transposons.

In contrast to the CG suppression seen in the mammalian genome, there are small regions of DNA 300–3000 bp in length where the frequency of CpGs is at either expected values or higher. These areas are known as CpG islands and they are protected from methylation. CpG islands represent roughly 1–2% of the genome, and are located close to the promoter regions of roughly half of all human genes (Antequera et al., 1990). The methylation of promoters and internal CpG sites silence the gene with which it is associated. This occurs in the promoters of selected genes and on the inactivated X-chromosome of females. It also plays a role in genomic imprinting, whereby genes are expressed differently on maternal and paternal chromosomes as a result of differences in DNA methylation between the parental alleles (Reik and Walter, 2001). This silencing is permanent and transmitted through mitosis (Baylin et al., 2000).

Apart from some exceptions, CpG islands located in the promoter or the inside of active genes should be unmethylated. This is why aberrant methylation in the promoters of normally active genes has an important role in loss-of-gene function. The first two genes shown to have aberrant CpG island promoter methylation in cancer were the gene for calcitonin (CALCA) and *MyoD*. Since then, CpG island methylation in other tumour suppressor genes known to be involved in cancers have been observed in genes such as E-cadherin, *hMLH1*, *BRCA*-1, *pRb*, $p16^{Ink4a}$ and $p14^{ARF}$ (Baylin and Herman, 2000).

The consequences of methylation are known, but the exact mechanism responsible in aberrant methylation is poorly understood. The main DNA methyltransferase enzyme DNMT1 works during DNA replication by recognizing methylated CpG sites on the parent strand and methylates correlating cytosines on the daughter strand. This enzyme, or other enzymes that work in a similar manner, may be functioning incorrectly in certain cancer cells (Rhee et al., 2000) (Figure 6.4).

Unlike genetic mutation, inactivation of a gene by promoter methylation is potentially reversible by demethylating drugs. Compounds based on the demethylating agent 5-aza-2'-deoxycytidine (Decitabine) may form the basis of a new class of anti-cancer drugs in methylation-positive tumours.

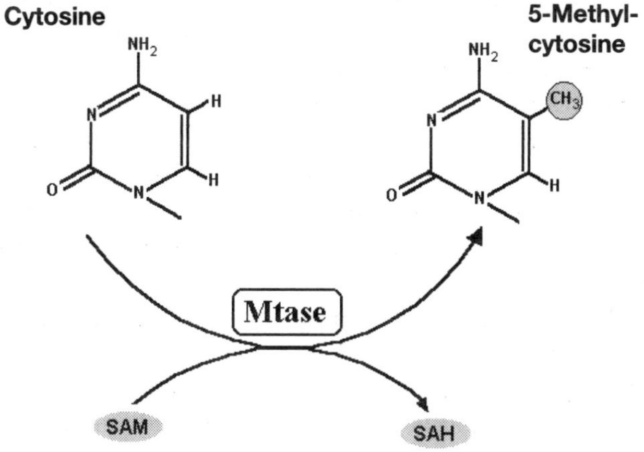

Figure 6.4 The DNA methyltransferase enzyme catalysing the addition of a methyl (CH_3) group on to a cytosine base, and using S-adenosyl methionine (SAM) as a methyl donor. SAH, S-adenosyl homocysteine.

Identifying cancer genes

There are many ways to identify the genetic abnormalities that develop during the progression of a cancer. Chromosomal loss, rearrangements and deletions of smaller regions of the chromosome give clues to the locations of many of the abnormal genes involved in carcinogenesis. Candidate tumour suppressor genes in these regions can then be screened for inactivating mutations or methylation.

Defining chromosomal abnormalities in a tumour

Karyotyping is used to count chromosome numbers, and to see large chromosomal alterations such as rearrangements and deletions. In karyotyping chromosomes are analysed by culturing the tumour cells, adding the drug colchicine, and staining and photographing the now visible chromosomes (Jorde et al., 2000). To detect much smaller deletions and abnormalities, other more sensitive techniques are used. These include fluorescence in situ hybridization (FISH) and comparative genomic hybridization (CGH).

In FISH a labelled chromosome-specific segment is hybridized with chromosomal DNA and visualized under a fluorescence microscope. This technique can tell whether there is a chromosomal deletion, because the labelled probe will not be able to hybridize. FISH can also distinguish whether there is deletion of a single chromosome, or if there is an additional chromosome segment, because it is possible to visualize how many locations the probe hybridizes (Trask, 1991). The use of differently coloured probes has led to several variations of this technique.

With CGH, tumour DNA and normal DNA are labelled with different colours and then hybridized together. Regions of the tumour DNA with deletions or duplications that are not present in the normal DNA will give a different colour balance, allowing the detection of multiple abnormal chromosomal regions (Kallioniemi et al., 1992).

Another method of screening for small areas of chromosomal imbalance is to do allelic imbalance analysis. In this technique highly variable repeat markers in the chromosomal region of interest, known as microsatellites, are screened in both tumour and normal tissue. If one of the heterozygous markers (multiple repeats) becomes homozygous (a single repeat) in the tumour, this suggests that an allele has been lost, and there is a deletion in this region. This is known as loss of heterozygosity (LOH) or allelic loss. Alleles can also be gained in the case of chromosomal duplications.

Mutational analysis

To detect relatively large deletions in a gene, Southern blotting is usually used. In this technique a labelled DNA probe is hybridized to a DNA fragment of interest that has been transferred to a nylon membrane (Southern, 1975). To screen for deletions under 50 bp in size and other small genetic alterations, the most sensitive way of screening genes of interest for mutations is direct DNA sequencing. Screening of multiple genes in many tumour samples is technically demanding, costly and time-consuming, so pre-screening techniques are usually used to pick out a sample that definitely contains a mutation. The region of interest has to be amplified up using a technique known as polymerase chain reaction (PCR).

Polymerase chain reaction

Polymerase chain reaction is a rapid and versatile method for amplifying a defined target DNA sequence within a source of DNA. Some prior knowledge of the DNA sequence of the target is needed and, from this sequence information, two oligonucleotide primers are designed that will hybridize to this sequence and surround the area to be amplified. When the DNA template is denatured (heated to form single-stranded DNA) these primers anneal and bind to the specific complementary DNA sequences at the target site. In the presence of a heat-resistant DNA polymerase enzyme and DNA precursor nucleotides, these primers can initiate the synthesis of new DNA strands, which are complementary to the DNA strands of the target DNA. PCR is a chain reaction, because the newly synthesized DNA acts as a template for further DNA synthesis in subsequent cycles. After about 25 cycles of DNA synthesis the products of the PCR will include about 10^5 copies of the specific target sequence. The PCR products can then be visualized using agarose gel electrophoresis. This technique uses the fact that, as DNA is a charged molecule, it can migrate through a porous gel when a current is passed through it. This allows DNA fragments to be separated according to size.

Pre-screening techniques

After amplifying an area of interest in the gene using PCR, the PCR products can be screened for genetic alterations using techniques such as SSCP (single-strand conformational polymorphism), DGGE (denaturing gradient gel electrophoresis) or DHPLC (denaturing high-performance liquid chromatography) analysis. SSCP and DGGE are both gel-based techniques, using the fact that certain conditions alter the rate of migration of DNA fragments in gel electrophoresis. DHPLC uses a similar technique, but DNA fragments are instead separated on a HPLC column and detected using computer software (Xiao and Oefner, 2001).

Genetic screening of cancer

As cancer has a strong genetic basis, genetic screening should have potential applications for determining prognostic information. In classic monogenic (one-gene) familial genetic disorders such as Huntington's disease, screening of potentially affected family members can allow people to know what their chances are of developing a disease. Screening can also allow potential parents to know what the likelihood is of any future offspring developing the condition. Unfortunately in cancer studies this is not as straightforward, as a result of the complexity of cancer genetics. Inherited cancer syndromes that act similarly to classic genetic diseases cause only about 1% of human cancer. A further 5–10% of all cancers (depending on how strictly defined) have a more general familial basis (Ponder, 2001). In these families several cases of common cancers are found, usually falling into general groups of cancers (e.g. breast and ovary, or colon, endometrium and urinary). Only these rarer familial cancers have a potential requirement for genetic screening. If the risk to a family member can be determined, there is a possibility that preventive steps can be taken.

So far, the only major familial cancer screened for is familial breast and ovarian cancer caused by the genes *BRCA*-1 and *BRCA*-2. Some cancer centres now offer screening for *BRCA*-1 and *BRCA*-2 mutations in families with multiple cases of these tumours. If mutations are found it is estimated that a woman has up to an 85% lifetime risk of developing breast cancer and a 60% risk of developing ovarian cancer (Armstrong et al., 2000). If *BRCA* mutations are detected, intensive monitoring can be used to pick up developing tumours at an early stage. For the most high-risk cases preventive measures such as prophylatic mastectomy, or taking drugs that reduce the chances of these cancers (such as tamoxifen), can be considered. Unfortunately *BRCA*-1 and *BRCA*-2 mutation-associated familial cases account for only around 15–20% of familial cancers, so possibly there are many genetic risk factors yet to be discovered (Balmain, 2001). Genes that confer strong susceptibility to other familial cancers may eventually be screened in a similar manner. Useful genes for which screening programmes may be developed could include the $p16^{Ink4a}$ gene in familial skin melanoma, and the various tumour suppressor and DNA-repair genes involved in the familial colon cancer syndromes, familial adenomatous polyposis (FAP) and hereditary non-polyposis colon cancer (HNPCC).

Future applications of cancer genetics: chemosensitivity and gene therapy

Aside from the applications of genetic screening in the small number of familial cancers, genetic technologies will have more and more applications in the research and treatment of cancer. By defining the genetic abnormalities and alterations in specific types of cancer, we have massively increased our understanding of how these tumours develop, helping us to understand how to target and fight them, and at the same time discovering new drug targets. The closer that specific tumour cells have been studied, the more genetic abnormalities and differences in their genetic profile have been discovered, even in cells that are supposedly from the same tumour type. Techniques such as DNA microchips are allowing us simultaneously to profile many of the genetic changes from tumour to tumour. The more we understand how certain tumours with certain molecular profiles behave, the more we will be able specifically to tailor treatments for them. Eventually we will be able to tailor specific drug regimens for specific tumours, minimizing drug resistance and side effects.

Ultimately the best way of treating a cancer would be to find a way of genetically modifying the tumour cells, correcting the genetic defect. This technique is known as 'gene therapy', and currently much research is going into potential mechanisms for delivering genes to target cells, inhibiting the expression of specific genes and correcting genetic defects. This technology is a still a long way from becoming a useful clinical treatment, but has such great potential for the future that it has to be discussed here. There have been several potential gene delivery systems discovered to date, and potential vectors currently being studied include attenuated DNA and RNA viruses that integrate part of their genome (containing the target gene) into a target cell. These viruses have had most of their viral genes removed to stop them replicating, but there are still safety and immunological problems with the technique. Non-viral vectors that avoid these problems are also currently in development, including liposome vector systems, but these have a lower efficiency of gene transfer and do not integrate genes into the chromosome, so gene expression is for a shorter duration (Strachan and Read, 1999).

Recessive monogenic disorders are the most amenable diseases to be treated with this technique, because only small amounts of introduced gene product can potentially have an effect. Trials have been carried out on diseases including adenosine deaminase deficiency (ADA), cystic fibrosis and familial hypercholesterolaemia. The use of gene therapy technologies to treat cancers is potentially more complicated, because a cancer cell can have several different genes mutated. Tumour cells are constantly being selected against, and evolve resistance to, various treatments, so similar problems would need to be overcome if this technique was used as a cancer therapy. Different strategies have been tested in cancers including pancreatic cancer (Halloran et al., 2000). Strategies have included the addition of copies of working tumour suppressor genes, and techniques that attempt to enable targeted cell death. This works by the genetic introduction into the tumour of an enzyme that can convert non-toxic drug precursors into toxic forms that will selectively kill the tumour cells without any side effects. More research is needed to improve the targeting of this technology, and increase the efficiency, gene uptake and safety, but despite these problems gene therapy has enormous potential for the future of medicine.

CHAPTER 7

The immune system

HELMOUT MODJTAHEDI AND AILSA CLARKE

Background

Our body is constantly insulted by a variety of pathogens such as bacteria, viruses, fungi and parasites from the environment. These pathogens are different in shape and size (e.g. from 20 nm [viruses] up to 7 m [tapeworm]) and can cause infectious disease and cancer in different ways. Our body has evolved three kinds of defence strategy against these foreign invaders and other antigens: (1) physical (e.g. intact skin and mucosa) and chemical (e.g. acid in stomach) barriers; (2) natural (also called innate or non-specific) immune responses (e.g. phagocytosis); and (3) adaptive (also called acquired or specific) immune responses. In most cases, the penetration of pathogens into our body and their consequent destruction may be achieved successfully by the first two lines of body defences. If not, the pathogens can multiply and disease ensues and the body recovers as a result of activation of the adaptive response against the invading pathogens (Figure 7.1). The adaptive immune response against pathogens is mediated by a special group of immune cells called lymphocytes. The activation, proliferation and differentiation of different types of lymphocytes can result in the elimination of such pathogens by the antibody-mediated immune (AMI) response or cell-mediated immune (CMI) response. More importantly, once the infection is cleared, most of the expanded population of antigen-specific lymphocytes undergo programmed cell death, whereas a small number of these lymphocytes differentiate into long-lived memory lymphocytes, which remain in the circulation for decades after the first exposure to that particular pathogen. As a result, when the body encounters the same pathogen a second time, these pathogens are destroyed very rapidly (within hours) and more efficiently by activation of the memory cells. In such situations, the individual is said to have developed immunity or specific resistance against that particular pathogen. Obviously, the pathogens have also developed

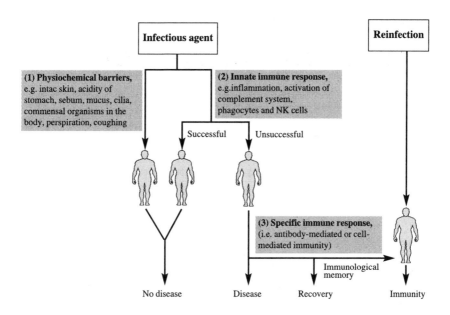

Figure 7.1 Three different strategies used by the body against foreign pathogens. The first two lines of defence are usually sufficient to eliminate infectious agents. If not, the body recovers as a result of activation of the adaptive immune responses, which generate specific populations of lymphocytes against the invading pathogens. Some of these lymphocytes remain in circulation as memory cells and provide immunity against re-infection by the original antigen. The principle of immunization is to alter the antigen in a way that prevents it causing disease but stimulates production of memory B or T lymphocytes against such antigens. NK, natural killer.

various strategies (e.g. by mutation, downregulation of immunogenic antigens) to overcome the body's defences. So it is a constant battle between the invader and the host.

In addition to their prime role in fighting infectious agents, it is clear that the immune system plays an important role in a number of pathological conditions, e.g. abnormal immune responses against a harmless substance (e.g. food, pollen) or self-antigens have been associated with allergies and autoimmune diseases. In contrast, normal immune responses against a tissue or organ transplantation from an incompatible individual are associated with transplant rejection (Buckley, 2003). The immune cells in transplanted organs and tissues may also attack and destroy the tissues of the host causing graft-versus-host disease (Gulbahce et al., 2003).

There are convincing lines of evidence that suggest that a fully functional immune system can prevent the incidence of cancer, e.g. cancer incidence together with infectious diseases increase rapidly in old age (see Chapter 1) as the ability of the immune system to recognize and provoke a strong immune response against pathogens declines (Franceschi et al., 2000; Effros, 2003). In addition, the incidence of cancer has been shown to be increased in immunosuppressed patients such as those treated with cytotoxic drugs and those with AIDS (acquired immune deficiency syndrome) (Appay and Rowland-Jones, 2002; Vial and Descotes, 2003).

In general, as cancer cells are almost identical to other healthy body cells, the immune system is less efficient at dealing with tumours than with infectious agents. Indeed, most human antigens are tumour-associated antigens and are expressed in lower amounts in normal cells. In recent years, as a result of our better understanding of the cells and molecules of the immune system, the identification and characterization of tumour antigens of biological and clinical significance, and the development of novel adjuvants, we have been able to manipulate the immune system and provoke immune responses against human tumour antigens that are not normally immunogenic in cancer patients. Several clinical trials are currently under way in cancer patients using tumour cells that have been transfected with genes for cytokines and other co-stimulatory molecules, tumour antigens or antigen fragments in combination with new adjuvants as the source of cancer vaccines (Moingeon, 2001; Romero et al., 2002). Monoclonal antibodies have been developed against human tumour antigens and some of these antibodies are currently used for the management of human cancers (see Chapter 9).

In this chapter, a detailed account of the cells and molecules of the normal immune system is presented together with their functions. The relationship between the immune system and cancer, novel immunotherapeutic strategies (e.g. cancer vaccines) for human cancers, together with the effects of cytotoxic drugs on the immune system, are then discussed.

The first line of body defence

As mentioned above, our body has evolved three kinds of defence strategy against infectious agents, some of which (i.e. viruses) have been associated with the development of human cancers (Tortora and Grabowski, 2003; see also Chapter 2). All viruses, and some bacteria, can live and multiply inside the host cells and are called intracellular pathogens. In contrast, most bacteria and larger parasites live and multiply outside the host cells in the body tissues and fluids, and are called extracellular pathogens. The first line of defence against infectious agents is non-immunological and involves a number of physical and chemical barriers, also known as external defences. An unbroken skin is the most important protection for the body and acts as a physical barrier to stop invasion by foreign micro-organisms and other substances. The skin also has normal secretions such as acidic sweat and fatty acids from oil glands which can destroy or inhibit bacterial growth on its surface. In addition, there is also a normal population of microflora that can colonize the surface of the skin and inhibit growth of potential pathogens by competing for the available space and nutrients at the site (Wood, 2001).

The mucous membranes at the openings to the digestive, respiratory, urinary and reproductive tracts also protect the body from invasion by foreign micro-organisms. Mucus traps bacteria or other foreign substances and can be expelled from the body. The urinary and reproductive tracts are free from micro-organisms under normal circumstances. Regular urination and secretion of mucus flushes any micro-organisms towards the outside of the body, although some microflora or opportunistic pathogens can enter from the surrounding areas. Movement of the gut contents and expulsion of the faeces helps to remove unwanted bacteria. Other physical and chemical barriers include the antimicrobial enzyme lysozyme in perspiration, tears, saliva and nasal secretions, and the acidity of gastric juice in the stomach (Wood, 2001; Tortora and Grabowski, 2003). Such physical and chemical barriers may be sufficient in preventing the infection and disease caused by pathogens (see Figure 7.1, page 75).

The immune system is a complex network of immune cells, cytokines, lymphoid tissues and organs that work together to eliminate infectious agents and other antigens (Tables 7.1–7.3). When infectious agents are not stopped by the physical and chemical barriers described above, they enter the body through the skin or mucous membranes. This in turn initiates the first line of immunological defence called the innate, non-specific or natural immune response. If the pathogens are not eliminated by the innate immune response, disease ensues and the body recovers as a result of activation of the adaptive response, or specific or acquired immune response (see Figure 7.1). The two important differences between the innate and adaptive immune response are that the latter is highly specific for a particular pathogen/antigen and the response improves with each subsequent exposure to the same antigen. However, as we see later, both innate and adaptive immune responses work together at several levels (e.g. by releasing growth-promoting cytokines) to destroy the invading antigens.

Innate (natural, non-specific) immune response

The innate immune response is present at birth and is mediated by a complex sequence of cellular and molecular events including phagocytosis, inflammation, complement activation and natural

Table 7.1 Cells of the immune system

Cells	Functions
Phagocytes	Immune cells that can ingest and digest foreign antigens/pathogens by the process of phagocytosis, e.g. macrophages, neutrophils
Antigen-presenting cells	Process and present antigens to T lymphocytes, e.g. dendritic cells, macrophages, B cells
Natural killer cells	Kill tumour cells and some viral infected cells. Are lymphocytes but, unlike B and T cells, lack specificity and memory
B lymphocytes	Express antibodies on their cell surface which can bind to antigens and differentiate to antibody-producing plasma cells
Plasma cells	The antibody-secreting form of B lymphocytes
Cytotoxic T cell (killer T cell, Tc)	Subset of T lymphocytes (CD8$^+$) that recognize cells expressing foreign antigens in association with MHC-I molecules, and kill by releasing the cytokines perforin and lymphotoxin. Releases other cytokines that stimulate phagocytosis and inhibit viral replication
T-helper cell (Th, T4)	Subset of T lymphocytes (CD4$^+$) which produces cytokines that stimulates both antibody-mediated and cell-mediated immune response
Memory T cells	Develop after the first exposure to a particular antigen. Remains in circulation and recognizes the original antigen years after the first exposure; responds more rapidly and efficiently in second and subsequent exposures
Suppressor T cells	Downregulate the immune responses

Table 7.2 Important cytokines of the immune system

Cytokine	Function
Interleukin	
IL-1	Mainly from macrophages, contributing to fever and T-cell and macrophage activation
IL-2	Secreted by T-helper cells. Co-stimulates proliferation of T-helper cells, cytotoxic T cells and B cells. Activates natural killer (NK) cells
IL-4	Produced by T and B cells and macrophages. Involved in activation of B cells, differentiation of T-helper 2 (Th2) cells and suppression of Th1 cells

Table 7.2 (Cont.)

Cytokine	Function
IL-8	Macrophage-derived chemoattractant for immune system cells and phagocytes to site of inflammation
IL-10	Secreted by T and B cells and macrophages. Involved in suppression of macrophage function and Th1 cells. Activates B cells
IL-12	Produced mainly by dendritic cells and macrophages. Mainly involved in differentiation of Th1 cells and activation of NK cells and T cells
Interferons (IFNs)	Produced by macrophages, lymphocytes and NK cells. A major macrophage activator. Activates NK cells. Enhances antibody-mediated immune (AMI) and cell-mediated immune (CMI) responses. Antiviral activity
Tumour necrosis factor (TNF)	Mainly from macrophages and T-helper cells. Cytotoxic to tumour cells. Enhances activity of phagocytic cells
Lymphotoxin (LT)	Secreted by cytotoxic T cells. Kills cells by activating cell's own caspase enzymes which induce an endonuclease to degrade the cell's DNA (apoptosis)
Perforin	Secreted by cytotoxic T cells and NK cells. Polymerizes to form tubular structures, which perforate the lipid bilayer of the target cells leading to osmotic lysis
Granzymes	Secreted by cytotoxic T cells and NK cells. Pass through perforin pores and induce apoptosis from within the target cell cytoplasm
Transforming growth factor (TGFβ)	Produced by T cells and monocytes. Inhibits T- and B-cell proliferation and NK cell activity

Table 7.3 Important recognition moieties of the immune system

	Function
Antibodies	Produced by plasma cells differentiated from B lymphocytes. Enhance phagocytosis by opsonization. Neutralize antigens and activate complement. The antigen–antibody complex can bind to effector cells such as natural killer (NK) cells and macrophages targeting the antigen for destruction by antibody-dependent cell-mediated cytotoxicity (ADCC)
Complement	Over 20 serum glycoproteins which once activated lead to cell lysis, inflammation and opsonization

Table 7.3 (Cont.)

	Function
MHC	Major histocompatibility complex (MHC) molecules bind and 'present' antigenic peptides on the surfaces of cells for recognition by the antigen-specific T-cell receptor (TCR). Two classes: MHC-I on all nucleated cells, MHC-II on antigen-presenting immune cells
CD4	Molecules expressed on T-helper cells bind antigenic peptides presented by MHC-II
CD8	Molecules expressed on cytotoxic T cells bind antigenic peptides presented by MHC-I
Co-stimulatory molecules	Adhesion molecules/cytokines which provide the second signal for T-cell activation
Antigens/Epitopes	Substances that provoke immune responses (e.g. bacteria, pollen, transplanted tissues) are called antigens. Each antigen may have several components called epitopes and each epitope provokes the production of a specific antibody or stimulates a specific T lymphocyte (antigen = antibody generator)
Vaccine	A modified form of the original antigen that is used in immunization in order to stimulate the production of memory B cells and memory T cells without causing the disease. Antigenic preparation that is used in educating the immune system
Chemotaxis	The migration of a cell to the site of infection in response to a chemical stimulus (e.g. complement components) causing accumulation of leukocytes in inflamed tissues

killer (NK) cell activation. In contrast to the adaptive immune response, which improves with each successive exposure to the same antigen, the innate immune response is non-specific so does not change after repeated exposure to the same antigen. Some of the main components of the innate immune system, also called innate immunity, are described briefly here.

Phagocytosis and phagocytic cells

Phagocytosis is a multistep process by which phagocytic cells engulf and destroy infectious agents. As with other types of white blood cells, phagocytic cells are derived from a common pluripotent stem cell in the red bone marrow (Table 7.1). Phagocytes are attracted to the site of infection by a process called **chemotaxis**. Examples of chemotactic factors include microbial products, damaged leukocytes or tissue cells, complement components (e.g. C5a) and certain cytokines. The process continues with **adherence** of the phagocyte's plasma membrane to the surface of the micro-organism. This occurs more readily after opsonization where the microbe is coated by complement proteins or antibody molecules (see below). By extending the plasma membrane projections, called pseudopodia, phagocytic cells engulf the pathogen forming a phagocytic vacuole (i.e. phagosome) and fuse it with a lysosome. The phagocytosed pathogen can then be **digested** by the appropriate digestive enzymes and bactericidal chemicals. The indigestible products are ejected from the cell by **exocytosis**. Examples of phagocytic cells include neutrophils, monocytes and macrophages.

Neutrophils, which are the most abundant type of white blood cell, respond very rapidly to infection and are relatively short-lived (1–5 days); they can phagocytose only small pathogens such as viruses and bacteria. In response to infection, bone marrow can produce between 1 and 2×10^{11} neutrophils per day, and the number of neutrophils in the circulation does not alter with age (Lords et al., 2001). In contrast to neutrophils, macrophages (big eaters) in the tissues are derived from monocytes in the blood and respond more slowly to chemotactic stimuli than neutrophils, but are more efficient in the phagocytosis of the remaining living and dead pathogens. Macrophages can live for months or years and kill infectious agents by several mechanisms, e.g. the secretion of a wide range of molecules such as antiviral interferon or antibacterial lysozyme, and generation of oxygen radicals, nitric oxide and chlorine-containing products (Wood, 2001). Macrophages may be fixed in a particular tissue (e.g. Kupffer cells in the liver, microglia in the brain) or they may move throughout the body in search of pathogens (termed 'wandering macrophages'). The activated macrophages produce a number of cytokines (e.g. interleukin-1 [IL-1], IL-8, tumour necrosis factor α [TNFα] and interferon-α [IFN-α]), which stimulate an inflammatory response and bring an additional army of immune cells and molecules to the site of infection (Table 7.2). This additional array of cells and molecules can in turn destroy the invading pathogens more effectively.

Macrophages are also very important in the activation of adaptive (specific) immune responses against invading pathogens by presenting a fragment of processed antigen on their cell surface in association with major histocompatibility complex (MHC) class II molecules to CD4$^+$ T lymphocytes (see later). This results in the activation of CD4$^+$ T-helper lymphocytes which in turn can stimulate both the antibody-mediated and cell-mediated immune responses against infectious agents (Figure 7.2).

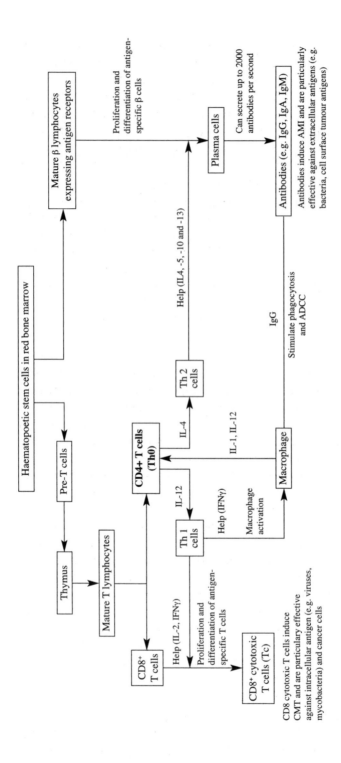

Figure 7.2 The central role played by CD4+ T-helper cells in all types of immune responses. The CD4+ T cells stimulated by antigen differentiate into CD4+ T-helper cell subsets Th1 and Th2. The cytokine released by Th1 cells in turn helps the cell-mediated immune response by increasing the population of antigen-specific CD8+ cytotoxic T cells and by activating macrophages that are important in the innate immune response. The cytokines released by Th2 cells can aid the antibody-mediated immune response by increasing the population of antigen-specific B cells and plasma cells. The production of cytokines by macrophages can also activate the proliferation and differentiation of T-helper cells. AMI, antibody-mediated immunity; CMI, cell-mediated immunity; IFN, interferon; IL, interleukin.

Inflammation

Damage to the body's tissues by microbial infection, physical agents such as heat or sharp objects, or chemical agents such as acid burns lead to a complex series of non-specific physiological responses called inflammation. The main aims are to localize the infection and prevent the spread of any microbial invaders, to recruit additional immune cells (e.g. neutrophils, monocytes) and molecules from the blood to the infected area, to neutralize toxins and to repair and replace damaged tissue. The tissue macrophages can stimulate inflammation further by releasing cytokines (IL-1, IL-8 and TNFα) that cause vasodilatation and increased vascular permeability, and are chemotactic for neutrophils and monocytes (Wood, 2001). Vasodilatation increases blood flow to the damaged area, leading to redness and heat at the site of injury. This allows an increase in the concentration of complement and other chemotactic factors to the infected areas which ultimately enhances phagocyte migration and phagocytosis at the site of injury. Tissue repair can then occur once all harmful substances and damage have been removed.

Complement activation

Another component of the innate immune response is the activation of the complement system. The complement system contains a cascade of inactive proteins in the blood that can be activated after the binding of an antibody to bacteria and other foreign cells or an alternative pathway. Once activated, the complement system generates a number of biologically active proteins that enhance inflammation, promote cell lysis and enhance phagocytosis by oponization. For example, the complement proteins C3a, C4a and C5a enhance inflammatory reactions by dilatation of arteries, release of histamine from mast cells and basophils, and attraction of neutrophils by chemotaxis. Other members of the complement system promote cell lysis by forming the membrane attack complex (C5b–C6, C7, C8 and C9). The complement fragment C3b is also an important opsonin and can coat the cell surface of pathogens. Phagocytic cells such as macrophages, monocytes and neutrophils all have C3b receptors on their surface. Such receptors can in turn help the elimination of the pathogens by promoting phagocytosis (Reeves and Todd, 2000; Wood, 2001; Tortora and Grabowski, 2003).

Natural killer cells

Natural killer cells are a distinct subpopulation of lymphocytes that play an important role in the natural immune response by mediating cytotoxic effects in the target cells and by releasing cytokines such as

IFNγ and TNFα (see Tables 7.1 and 7.2). Unlike B or T lymphocytes, NK cells lack specificity and memory but can induce spontaneous lysis of cells infected by viruses and various tumour cells by secretion of perforin and other lytic enzymes (Solana and Mariani, 2000). As described in Chapter 9, NK cells, in addition to their direct cytotoxic killing, can induce an antibody-dependent cell-mediated cytotoxicity (ADCC) in target cells by binding to the Fc portion of the antibody, e.g. organisms such as protozoa or helminths that are too large to be engulfed by phagocytic cells can be coated by antibodies. When the antigen-binding sites of the antibody (e.g. human IgG1 and IgG3 antibodies) have bound to such antigens, the Fc portion of the antibody is free and can bind to the Fc receptor on NK cells and direct cell killing by ADCC (see Figure 7.2). In addition to NK cells, macrophages, neutrophils and eosinophils also have Fc receptors that can bind to the Fc portion of the antibody molecule and direct cell killing by ADCC.

Although the absolute number of NK cells increases with age, their cytotoxic capacity decreases and this is a characteristic feature of immunosenescence (Malaguarnera et al., 2001), e.g. NK cells from old donors have been shown to respond less efficiently to the mitogenic cytokine IL-2 and this can result in decreased proliferation of NK cells and decreased production of IFN by NK cells. This may ultimately lead to a decreased cytotoxic response by NK cells against the target antigen on the infectious agent or tumour cell (Solana and Mariani, 2000).

Cytokines

Both natural and adaptive immunity are coordinated by about 60 cytokines (Tagawa, 2000; Sprent and Surh, 2003). These are small protein hormones that can stimulate or inhibit many normal cell functions but are less specific and more localized than endocrine hormones (see Table 7.2). Cytokines can be divided into several families including interleukins, interferons, tumour necrosis factors, colony-stimulating factors and chemokines, which regulate the migration of cells between and within tissues, e.g. there are around 22 different interleukins numbered 1–22. Of these, IL-1 is secreted by macrophages and monocytes and can stimulate an inflammatory response and activate lymphocytes (see Table 7.2 and Figure 7.2). IL-2 is produced by T-helper lymphocytes and stimulates the proliferation of T-helper (Th) cells, cytotoxic T cells and B lymphocytes, and activates NK cells. On the other hand, IL-10 and transforming growth factor-β (TGFβ) are immunosuppressants and inhibit the cytotoxic response of the immune system (T cells and macrophages) against the antigens from tumours and infectious agents (see Table 7.2; Levings et al., 2002). Therefore, drugs that block the immunosuppressive action of IL-10 and

TGFβ on the immune system may play an important role in the treatment of human cancers, whereas those that stimulate their function are useful in suppressing pathological immune responses such as in autoimmune diseases, allergies and transplantation rejection.

Some of the cytokines are listed in Table 7.2 together with their functions.

Adaptive (acquired, specific) immune response

In many situations, the non-specific immune responses described above (e.g. phagocytosis, NK cell activation, inflammation), with which we are born and that occur in the first few hours of infection, may be sufficient to overcome the pathogens. If not, disease can ensue and the body may recover after the activation of adaptive immune responses against the invading pathogens (see Figure 7.1). There are two types of adaptive immune responses, namely antibody-mediated immune (AMI) responses and cell-mediated immune (CMI) responses.

The most relevant cells in providing adaptive immune responses are lymphocytes, which make up between 25 and 35% of white blood cells; their total number in a healthy individual is close to one billion (10^{12}). Two major types of lymphocytes, called B cells and T cells, are present in the blood in a 1:5 ratio. B cells develop into mature immunocompetent cells in the red bone marrow and each B cell expresses an antigen receptor (i.e. antibody) of a single specificity on its cell surface and is responsible for the AMI response (see Figure 7.2). In AMI, the binding of antigen to antigen receptor (i.e. antibody) on B cells can result in the activation and differentiation of B cells into antibody-secreting plasma cells. However, to ensure full activation and differentiation of B cells into plasma cells in response to most antigens and antibody class switching (e.g. from low-affinity IgM subclass into high-affinity IgG subclass) requires a co-stimulator signal provided by the interaction of B cells with CD4$^+$ Th cells (i.e. T cells expressing CD4 antigen – see below). The binding of CD154 molecules on the CD4$^+$ T cell to CD40 molecules on the B cell, together with production of cytokines such as IL-4 and IL-5 by CD4$^-$ Th cells, can result in the full activation of B cells and their differentiation into antibody-producing plasma cells (see Figure 7.2).

Each plasma cell secretes up to 2000 antibodies per second against the original antigen and this process can continue for about 4–5 days. The antibody production by plasma cells can be increased by the cytokine IL-6. The secreted antibodies then circulate in the blood and lymphatic system, and bind to the original antigens, marking them for elimination by several mechanisms including: activation of the complement system, promotion of phagocytosis via opsonization, and mediation of ADCC with effector cells such as macrophages, NK cells and neutrophils (see Figure 7.2).

In contrast to the AMI response, a CMI response against the invading pathogen is mediated by T cells. Whereas B cells complete their maturation in the bone marrow, T lymphocytes develop from pre-T cells in the bone marrow and mature in the thymus into CD4$^+$- or CD8$^+$-expressing T cells (see Figure 7.2). In CMI, CD8$^+$ T cells recognizing the target antigen proliferate and differentiate into CD8$^+$ cytotoxic T cells (Tc) which kill the target antigens by delivering a lethal dose of the cytokines lymphotoxin and perforin or by directing apoptosis (see Figure 7.2). In contrast, T cells expressing CD4 antigen are called T-helper cells (Th0) and the binding of antigens to such cells results in their proliferation and differentiation into two CD4$^+$ Th cell subsets, Th1 and Th2. Th1 cells produce cytokines such as IL-2 and IFNγ which stimulate CMI responses against intracellular pathogens and tumour cells. In contrast, Th2 cells produce the cytokines IL-4, IL-5 and IL-6, which play a central role in regulating the AMI response against extracellular antigens and pathogens (see Figure 7.2). In addition, the production of cytokines by Th1 cells can enhance phagocytosis of the target antigen by macrophages of the innate immune system (see Figure 7.2). For this reason, CD4$^+$ helper T cells are viewed as the backbone of the immune system and their crucial role has been highlighted in patients with AIDS where the Th cells are targeted by the virus (Altfeld and Rosenberg, 2000). In a normal uninfected individual, the number of CD4$^+$ T cells is between 800 and 1200 cells/m^3 of blood. When the number of CD4$^+$ T cells falls below 200/mm^3 of blood towards the final stage of HIV infection, such individuals become particularly susceptible to opportunistic infections, caused by microbes that usually do not cause disease in healthy individuals, as well as cancers such as Kaposi's sarcoma and lymphomas. Indeed, AIDS is part of the evidence that supports the idea that immunosuppression can increase the incidence of cancer and the immune surveillance concept (Scadden, 2003; see below).

In addition to CD8$^+$ cytotoxic and CD4$^+$ Th cells, there are other populations of T lymphocytes that inhibit the immune response by releasing inhibitor cytokines; these cells are called suppressor T cells (Ts) (McHugh and Shevach, 2002).

MHC molecules, antigen recognition and processing in cell-mediated immunity

As described above, T lymphocytes are responsible for CMI responses against foreign antigens and the aim of most cancer vaccines under investigation or in development is to create antigen-specific, T-cell-mediated immune responses against tumour antigens.

However, as with B cells, successful activation of different T cells requires the presence of two signals, namely a recognition and a co-stimulatory signal. The first signal is recognition of the antigen by the antigen receptors on the surface of T cells, called T-cell receptors (TCRs), which results in the movement of the T cells from a resting phase of the cell cycle (i.e. G0) to G1 phase. However, unlike some B cells which can bind directly to an antigen with their unique antigen receptors (i.e. antibodies), the TCRs on both CD4$^+$ and CD8$^+$ T cells can recognize only a fragment of an antigen that has been processed and presented in association with a unique cell surface self-antigen called the major histocompatibility complex (MHC) antigen. There are two major types of self-MHC molecules which are also called human leukocyte antigens (HLAs). MHC class I molecules are found on all body cells except red blood cells and present the intracellular antigens to the TCRs on CD8$^+$ T cells. In contrast, MHC class II molecules are present only on the surface of antigen-presenting cells (APCs), such as macrophages, B lymphocytes and dendritic cells, and are important in the presentation of exogenous antigens to the TCRs on CD4$^+$ Th cells (Figure 7.3).

After the binding of the MHC–antigen fragment complex to the TCR, the T cells become activated only if they receive a second signal called a co-stimulatory signal. This second signal has been shown to be essential for full activation of T cells. Most co-stimulatory molecules are cell adhesion molecules that allow the two cells to adhere to one another for a longer period and result in sustained proliferation and differentiation of T cells (Figure 7.3), e.g. activation and differentiation of CD4$^+$ T cells into Th cells requires the binding of CD28 molecules on CD4$^+$ T cells to CD80/CD86 molecules present on APCs. This in turn results in the production of IL-2, IL-2 receptor expression, and cell cycle progression and proliferation of activated T cells. In contrast to CD4$^+$ Th cells, the full activation of cytotoxic T cells against the target cells is promoted by the binding of the CD2 molecule on CD8$^+$ T cells to the CD58 molecule on target cells and by the interaction of lymphocyte functional antigen 1 (LFA-1) on the T cell with the intercellular adhesion molecule 1 (ICAM-1) on the target cells. Recognition of the antigens by the antigen receptors on the lymphocyte, in the absence of co-stimulatory signals, results in the production of no cytokines, a state of immunological unresponsiveness called anergy, or even increased apoptosis (Frauwirth and Thompson, 2002). Indeed, deficiencies or abnormality in some of these components can help tumour cells to escape recognition and destruction by T cells (see below).

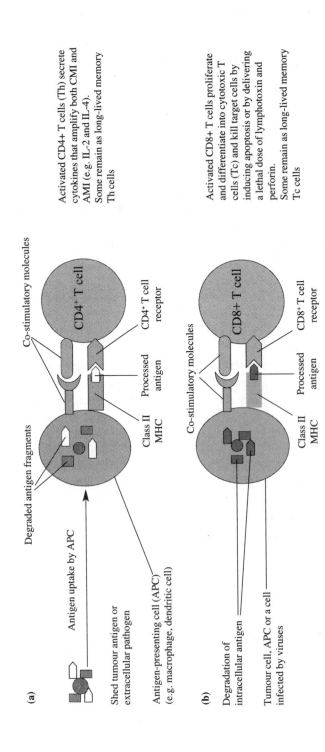

Figure 7.3 Successful activation of antigen-specific T-cell responses requires two signals: (a) CD4+ T-helper cells are activated only when the T-cell receptor (TCR) recognizes an antigen fragment, from exogenous antigens, in association with MHC-II molecules (signal 1) and receives a co-stimulatory signal by binding the CD28 molecule on T cells to a CD80/CD86 molecule on the antigen-presenting cell (signal 2). (b) CD8+ T cells are activated only when the TCR recognizes an antigen fragment, from endogenous antigens, in association with MHC-I molecule (signal 1) and receives a co-stimulatory signal via interaction between other cell surface (adhesions) molecules (signal 2). Recognition without the second signal results in anergy (i.e. a prolonged state of inactivity) and programmed cell death (apoptosis).

Adaptive immune system, immunological memory and immunization

Two characteristic features of the adaptive immune response are specificity for a particular antigen and immunological memory. Once the invading pathogens are destroyed by the adaptive immune response, some of the activated B and T lymphocytes differentiate into thousands of memory B and T cells. When the body encounters the same pathogen for a second time, these memory cells, which can remain in circulation for decades after the first exposure, increase their population so rapidly that the pathogens are destroyed before the individual develops any signs of disease (Sprent, 2003).

Indeed, the development of memory B and memory T cells against the antigen on the infectious agent or cancer cell is the rationale for successful immunization. The immunization of children against infectious agents is estimated to save the lives of 3 million children a year by helping the body to prevent primary infection (Andre, 2003). However, the development of vaccines against cancer is more challenging because, unlike vaccines against infectious diseases, cancer vaccines are developed for the treatment of disease that is already present in the body and not merely for its prevention (Berd, 1998; Moingeon, 2001).

In summary, the full activation of the immune system and successful destruction of any foreign antigens, cells and infectious agents by adaptive immune responses requires cooperation of immune cells of adaptive and innate immunity, the production of cytokines by such cells and the presence of co-stimulatory signals, which are essential for activation and proliferation of antigen specific B and T cells. Any abnormalities in one of the above components can lead to a state of immunological unresponsiveness against the target antigen.

The immune system and cancer

The interrelationship of immune response, old age and high incidence of cancer

In recent years several factors have been associated with the development of human cancers, including smoking, dietary factors, infectious agents (viruses and bacteria), chemicals, radiation and hereditary factors (see Chapter 2). The treatment of normal cells with these factors results in the mutation of a wide range of genes such as tumour suppressor genes or genes coding for growth factor, growth factor receptors, and motility and invasion factors. Such mutation can in turn result in malignant transformation of normal cells via the expression or release of either abnormal products or a high level of normal products (Hanahan and Weinberg, 2000).

As the incidence of cancer increases rapidly in old age, ageing is another important factor associated with human cancers. Around 65% of all cancers are diagnosed in people over the age of 65. Although the increasing accumulation of mutations in genes with time can be one factor that contributes to the high incidence of cancers in old age, recent evidence suggests that malfunction of the immune system may also contribute to the high incidence of cancers in elderly people (Burns and Leventhal, 2000; Ginaldi et al., 2001; Effros, 2003), e.g. it is well established that with increasing age there is deterioration of the immune response (i.e. immunosenescence) which results in increased susceptibility to infection, insufficient responses to vaccines and a high level of autoimmune disorders (Lords et al., 2001; Stacy et al., 2002). In particular, one of the common alterations in old age is a decline in T-cell-mediated immune responses. The decline in CMI with age is a multifactorial phenomenon and could be caused by: (1) a decrease in the population of naïve (resting) T lymphocytes with a concomitant increase in the population of antigen-specific memory T cells (i.e. exhaustion of immune resources); (2) the poor proliferative response of T cells to mitogens; and (3) a decrease in the expression of the co-stimulatory molecule (e.g. CD28) on T cells, together with an increase in the expression of the inhibitory molecule on CD4$^+$ Th cells (Franceschi et al., 2000; Appay and Rowland-Jones, 2002; Effros, 2003). Although there is no significant change in the AMI responses and the innate immune response is largely unchanged or even upregulated in old age, a decline in the T-cell-mediated immune response, such as that mediated by CD4$^-$ Th cells (see Figure 7.2), can reduce the overall immune response against cancer cells and therefore contribute to the high incidence of cancer in older people (Lords et al., 2001; Chen et al., 2002).

The immune surveillance theory

The immune surveillance theory put forward by Thomas in 1959 and redefined by Burnet (1967) states that the immune system is constantly patrolling the body for tumour (abnormal) cells, which are recognized as foreign, and mounts an immune response that results in their elimination before they become clinically detectable (Burnet, 1967). Although this concept remains controversial, a wide range of evidence supports it.

First, cancer patients with tumours infiltrated by many immune cells (e.g. proliferating CD8$^+$ T lymphocytes, macrophages, NK cells) have better survival than those with few infiltrated immune cells, suggesting that such immune cells are responsible for the improved survival in these patients (Ropponen et al., 1997; Naito et al., 1998; Nakano et al., 2001; Nakayama et al., 2002; Ohno et al., 2002). Second, as described above, the incidence of cancer is higher in older people and in the neonatal period when immune responses are less efficient. Third, the incidence of cancer is much higher in immunodeficient people (e.g. AIDS patients) than in those with a normal immune system. About 40% of HIV-infected individuals develop some form of cancer such as Kaposi's sarcoma (a malignant tumour of the blood vessels in the skin), or lymphoma (a malignant tumour of the lymphatic system) (Scadden, 2003). In addition, the incidence of certain types of cancer (e.g. skin cancers, lymphoma) is increased by four- to 500-fold in patients who have received organ transplants, whose immune systems have been downregulated with immunosuppressive drugs; reversal of the immunosuppression can result in tumour regression (Abgrall et al., 2002; Lutz and Heemann, 2003; Vial and Descotes, 2003). Furthermore, spontaneous regression of malignant tumours occurs in patients with melanoma, renal cell carcinoma, neuroblastoma, lymphoma and hepatocellular carcinoma, in whom the immune system plays an important role (Papac, 1998; Bromberg et al., 2002; Morimoto et al., 2002).

Mechanisms responsible for tumours escaping immune recognition

The proliferation and presence of clinically detectable tumours in cancer patients suggest that such tumours have been able to escape recognition and destruction by the immune system (i.e. the immune surveillance). From examination of sera and biopsies from cancer patients, it has become evident that cancer patients can produce both cell-mediated and antibody-mediated immune responses against tumour cells (Naito et al., 1998; Shimada et al., 2003). However, recent evidence suggests that the immune responses in some patients are either too weak to be effective in eliminating all tumours or, in other cases, too impaired to recognize the original tumours. Indeed, as explained in Chapter 9, the great majority of human tumour antigens are tumour-associated antigens; such antigens are also present in lower amounts on normal cells and are therefore less immunogenic (Kuroki et al., 2002). In addition, several other factors have been identified that can help the tumour cells to escape recognition and destruction by the immune system:

• Loss or downregulation of antigens recognized by tumour cells.
• Downregulation of MHC-I expression from the tumour cell's surface.

- Lack of co-stimulatory molecules (e.g. cytokines and adhesion molecules) which are necessary for T-cell activation.
- Overwhelming mass of tumour antigens and the presence of shed antigens in circulation.
- Increased level of immunosuppressive cytokines (TGFβ or IL-10).
- Downregulation of antigen-processing machinery.

In some situations, tumour cells escape immune recognition by losing or downregulating the expression of highly immunogenic antigens (Lollini and Forni, 2003). In other cases, tumour cells have been shown to lose or downregulate the expression of MHC-I molecules, which are essential (see Figure 7.2a) for antigen recognition and cell killing by CD8+ cytotoxic T cells (Natali et al., 1989; Paschin et al., 2003). In addition, antigen presentation by APCs to T cells in the absence of a co-stimulatory signal or mitogenic cytokines (e.g. IL-2) can result in immunological anergy. The release of immunosuppressive cytokines such as TGFβ and IL-10 by tumour cells and T cells can suppress the immune response against cancer cells, thus leading to tumour tolerance (Kirkbride and Blobe, 2003).

Immunotherapeutic strategies for human cancer

In recent years, as a result of better understanding of the immune system, including the mechanisms that are used by tumour cells to escape immune recognition and destruction and identification of novel antigens of biological and clinical significance at different stages of the cancer, immunotherapeutic approaches have been initiated in patients with a wide range of cancers (Berd, 1998; Armstrong and Hawkins, 2001; Costello et al., 2003; Waldman, 2003). The overall aim of such strategies is to provide protection against cancer cells, by either amplifying the immune response against cancer cells or correcting and breaking tolerance against tumour antigens via the patient's own immune system.

There are currently two main immunotherapeutic strategies against human cancers, namely the monoclonal antibody-based therapy of human cancer and the development of cancer vaccines. The former strategy has been described in detail in Chapter 9 and is particularly effective in the destruction of extracellular antigens, such as overexpressed HER-2 antigens in patients with metastatic cancer.

In recent years, several types of cancer vaccines have been prepared that are at different stages of clinical development including vaccines containing: (1) intact autologous tumour cells (derived from the patient to be treated) or intact allogeneic tumour cells (derived from other patients) modified by physical alteration, gene modification (with IL-2, granulocyte–macrophage colony-stimulating factor [GM-CSF]) or mixing with adjuvants (e.g. bacille Calmette-Guèrin [BCG] – an attenuated strain of *Mycobacterium bovis*, or QS-21, a material extracted from tree bark) that boosts the immune response against human tumour cells; (2) crude extracts of tumour cells; (3) purified extracts (e.g. gangliosides in melanoma); (4) peptides (MAGE proteins found in melanoma); (5) heat-shock proteins; (6) dendritic cells pulsed with tumour antigens and co-stimulatory molecules and cytokines; (7) DNA- and RNA-based vaccines; and (8) anti-idiotypic antibodies as surrogate antigens (Pardoll, 1998; Leitner et al., 2000; Berd, 2001; Lundqvist and Pisa, 2002; Davidson et al., 2002: Ehrke, 2003). The major aim of such strategies is to direct tumour killing by inducing cell-mediated (antigen-specific T cell), anti-tumour immune responses in such patients.

The potential of immunotherapeutic strategies for the treatment and prevention of human cancers has generated considerable excitement and interest among tumour immunologists and oncologists worldwide. In particular, the extraordinary capacity of dendritic cells to capture and process tumour antigens, together with their capacity to present the fragments of such antigens in association with MHC-I and MHC-II molecules to CD4$^+$ T cells and CD8$^+$, and therefore their activation, have made them ideal as a source of human cancer vaccines (Figure 7.4). The results of clinical trials with different type of vaccines should clarify the full potential and limitation of each strategy and would ultimately lead to the development of a more effective therapeutic strategy directed against a specific population of cancer patients (Tjoa et al., 1997; Bodey et al., 2000; Bremers et al., 2000; Romero et al., 2002; Sabel and Sondak, 2002; Boon and Van den Enbde, 2003; Ehrke, 2003).

Immune system in patients undergoing chemotherapy and radiotherapy

All the immune cells of our body (e.g. neutrophils, lymphocytes, monocytes, NK cells) are developed from stem cells in the bone marrow. In the bone marrow, there is about one stem cell for every 100 000 blood cells. Neutrophils, which are the largest fraction of white blood cells, account for about 54–63% of all white blood cells and they are the first immune cells to arrive at the site of infection and the first line of defence against invading pathogens. Their numbers in circulation do not change with age in normal individuals (see earlier). However, as they have a short half-life in the blood, the

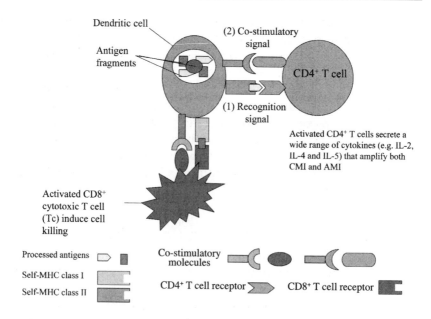

Figure 7.4 Therapeutic strategy using dendritic cells as source of cancer vaccine. Dendritic cells express high levels of both MHC-I and MHC-II molecules on their cell surface. They can be harvested from cancer patients, loaded with human tumour antigens, pulsed with co-stimulatory molecules and returned to patients. Such cells can then present the tumour antigen fragments in association with MHC-I to cytotoxic CD8+ T cells and therefore mediate tumour cell killing by cell-mediated immune (CMI) response. In addition some of the antigen processed by dendritic cells can be presented in association with MHC-II molecules to CD4+ T-helper cells, which secrete a wide range of cytokines that help cell killing via CMI and antibody-mediated immune (AMI) responses and activate macrophage cell killing (see Figure 7.2).

bone marrow produces about 10^{11} neutrophils a day. Likewise, as discussed above, lymphocytes are very important in mediating adaptive immune responses against both intracellular and extracellular antigens and cancer cells. About 1000 million lymphocytes die and are replaced by the stem cells in the bone marrow every day.

One of the common and most dangerous side effects associated with an intensive course of chemotherapy and/or radiotherapy is bone marrow suppression and a reduction in the number of white blood cells (leukocytes) in the blood, a condition called leukopenia (Kubota et al., 2001; Hood, 2003). In particular, febrile neutropenia is a common complication of cancer chemotherapy which can cause death in 4–21% of cancer patients (Young and Feld, 2000; Ray-Coquard et al., 2003). With the advances in genetic engineering, recombinant forms of haematopoietic cytokines, also called CSF, have been generated that stimulate the proliferation and differentiation of different populations of white blood cells, e.g. the human G-CSF filgrastim has been shown to be effective in reducing neutropenia, decreasing its severity and duration, reducing hospitalizations and the incidence of infection, and improving quality of life in patients undergoing chemotherapy (Valley, 2002). A modified version of filgrastim, called pegfilgrastim, has been developed that has a much longer serum half-life and therefore requires less frequent administration in patients undergoing aggressive forms of chemotherapy by reducing the risk of chemotherapy-induced neutropenia (Crawford, 2002; Hood, 2003).

Summary and future considerations

It is clear that a better understanding of our immune system and the way it can differentiate between self-antigens and non-self-antigens will have a huge impact on different areas of clinical medicine. Such developments could help treatment of patients with cancer, infection, autoimmune diseases and allergies, as well as those patients undergoing organ transplantation or requiring aggressive forms of chemo- or radiotherapy.

In relation to cancer, the identification of novel antigens not only plays a crucial role in the biology and pathology of different types of cancers but also activate both cell-mediated and antibody-mediated immune responses, a more effective immunotherapeutic strategy (i.e. cancer vaccines) for educating our immune system could be developed. In this way, persistent tumour antigens would be recognized and remembered by memory B and T cells already present in the immune system, leading to the prevention of most human cancers (Lollini and Forni, 2003). However, as discussed above, immunization against such persistent tumour antigens should be performed in young people when the immune system is most efficient at recognizing and destroying foreign antigens (Miller, 1996; Abgrall et al., 2002; Davidson et al., 2002; Costello et al., 2003; Lollini and Forni, 2003; Waldman, 2003). Recent advances in this direction may be imminent thanks to advances in tumour immunology, cell and molecular biology of cancer, and mapping of the human genome, together with recent technological advances in genetic engineering and development of monoclonal antibodies (see Chapter 9).

CHAPTER 8

Tumour markers

F. GUY GABRIEL

It is generally agreed that the first tumour marker to be discovered was the Bence Jones proteins, which were identified in 1846 in acidified urine of some cancer patients. Subsequently, Bence Jones proteins have been identified as monoclonal free light chains of immunoglobulins. Concentrations of Bence Jones proteins are found to be raised in more than 50% of patients with multiple myeloma (Kyle, 1975; Magdelenat, 1992; Thomas and Sweep, 2001).

Since 1846, other proteins, enzymes, isoenzymes, receptors, structural elements and hormones have been identified as tumour markers in blood and other body fluids (ascites, pleural effusions, faecal occult blood, etc.) of patients with growing tumours. Examples include acid phosphatase for prostate cancer, α-fetoprotein (AFP) for hepatoma and carcinoembryonic antigen (CEA) for colorectal cancer. However, it was not until the early 1960s that trace amounts of these secreted tumour markers had been measurable from body fluids by radioimmunoassay methods (Yalow and Berson, 1960; Miles and Hales, 1968a). Further advances in immunoassay technologies in the 1970s and 1980s, in particular the use of monoclonal antibodies (Köhler and Milstein, 1975), have helped identify many new tumour markers. The use of recombinant DNA and nonradioactive detection methods has led to the development of automated immunoassay systems.

In addition molecular techniques such as polymerase chain reaction (PCR) have enabled the Human Genome Project and the development of microarray DNA technology (gene chips) to identify the molecular signatures of cancer. These techniques may, in the future, identify new tumour markers that can be used in early detection of some cancers.

It has only been since the mid-1990s, after detailed analysis of all the published literature about tumour markers (including clinical trials) by various panels of experts at international, national and regional levels, that tumour markers have been fully validated for clinical use within evidence-based medicine. The findings of these multidisciplinary expert panels have been published as recommendations and guidelines, including:

- Tumor Marker Expert Panel (American Society of Clinical Oncology, 1996): clinical practice guidelines for the use of tumour markers in breast and colorectal cancer.
- Association of Clinical Biochemists in Ireland (1999): guidelines for the use of tumour markers.
- European Group for Tumor Markers (EGTM, 1999): consensus recommendations.
- Update (2000) of the recommendations for the use of tumour markers in breast and colorectal cancer: clinical practice guidelines of the American Society of Clinical Oncology (Bast et al., 2001).
- European Society for Medical Oncology (ESMO, 2001): ESMO minimum clinical recommendations for diagnosis, treatment and follow-up of ovarian cancer.

These guidelines have a tendency either to favour clinical aspects of care (e.g. surgery) or to focus on laboratory investigations for monitoring the disease through the measurement of tumour markers (Sturgeon, 2002). These recommendations and guidelines have resulted in only a handful of serum tumour markers being recommended for clinical use. Others are still being investigated in ongoing clinical trials.

Today, with the development of automated immunoassays, tumour markers can be routinely measured in clinical biochemistry laboratories rather than in specialist laboratories. Often they may be used as part of clinical diagnosis and/or staging, predicting cancer prognosis and clinical management (monitoring, guiding treatment) of an individual patient, and may give an indication that the patient's tumour is not responding to treatment, or may have metastasized and warrants further investigation.

What are tumour markers?

Events within a tumour's development are governed by genetic or epigenetic mechanisms and signalling pathways. These complex intracellular molecular pathways are not yet fully understood and nor is the mechanism by which the tumour cells control and co-opt the neighbouring non-neoplastic cells for tumour development in the process of tumorigenesis. Often, mutation of regulatory oncogenes such as *ras*, c-*myc* and *p53*, and their expressed proteins, can be found to have increased in most cancer cells. The process of carcinogenesis may be disrupted at any stage, which results in heterogeneity among tumours of the same type and also within the same tumour mass. This is a result of the tumour cell's intrinsic genetic instability (Hanahan and Weinberg, 2000).

Tumour markers are biological or molecular substances (protein, carbohydrates, hormones, etc.) that can be produced and attributed to the events in tumorigenesis. They may be produced by the tumour cells themselves, or by the body in response to the presence of cancer, or in certain benign conditions, e.g. dermatofibroma, benign prostatic hyperplasia and benign prostatic hypertrophy. Those produced intra-cellularly, or on the cell membrane (oestrogen receptor – ER) are detected by immunohistochemistry (IHC) on the tumour tissue. Those secreted into body fluids can be quantified by immunoassay methods. The production of tumour markers can result from:

- Unique genes expressed only in tumour cells (cancer antigen 125 – CA125).
- Abnormal or higher than normal expression of specific biochemi-cal substances (prostatic acid phosphate – PAP, β_2-microglobulin – β_2M; growth factors, cytokines) than found in normal cells.
- Expression of fetal antigens, normally expressed during embry-ological development, but not present in adult normal tissue – known as oncofetal antigens (AFP). This is reflected by the fact that the morphology of the cancer tissue on histological examina-tion often resembles embryonic tissue rather than normal adult differentiated tissue (Sell, 1991).

However, other markers that may also be found in some normal tissue, or benign conditions, are often referred to as tumour-associ-ated antigens.

Since 1988 the accepted definition of a tumour marker is:

Biochemical tumor markers are substances developed in tumor cells and secreted into body fluids in which they can be quantitated by non-invasive analyses. Because of a correlation between marker concentration and active tumor mass, tumor markers are useful in the management of cancer patients. Markers, which are available for most cancer cases, are addi-tional, valuable tools in patient prognosis, surveillance and therapy moni-toring, whereas they are presently not applicable for screening. Serodiagnostic measurements of markers should emphasize relative trends instead of absolute values and cut-off levels.

The Fifth International Conference on Human Tumour Markers held in Stockholm, Sweden in 1988 (Suresh, 2001)

As already mentioned these 'tumour' markers can be divided into two groups:

1. Tumour markers: tumour-specific glycoproteins and mucins expressed only in tumour cells (CA125, CA19-9).
2. Tumour-associated markers: oncofetal antigens, oncogenes, onco-proteins, carbohydrates, hormones, enzymes, cytokines, soluble receptors, growth factors, cellular markers – not tumour specific, but expressed in higher levels than in normal tissue (CEA, AFP, β_2M, p21 ras protein, vascular endothelial growth factor – VEGF).

Which marker to measure is determined by the tumour type and whether the marker levels are likely to change during the course of the disease. These markers fall into two categories (Fertig and Hayes, 2001):

1. Static: these tend to remain constant throughout the natural history of a cancer and are measured once. They may be used as a prognostic indicator. They are usually measured by IHC on tissue samples. Examples include oestrogen receptor in breast cancer, HER-2/neu (c-erbB-2) and mutant *p53*.
2. Dynamic: these reflect the activity of the tumour. Levels may respond to change in the tumour as a result of therapy, and may be useful in predicting the response. They are normally measured in blood and body fluids. Examples include CA125 and CA19-9.

To date, no tumour marker has yet been found to be specific and able to be detected early enough to be the sole indicator of cancer or for use in mass screening programmes (Sell, 1991; Suresh, 2001; Schilsky and Taube, 2002).

In establishing a cancer diagnosis, a number of appropriate tumour markers may be measured initially, in conjunction with other investigations, to assist in staging and grading of the tumour. Although tumour markers may play a valuable role as part of investi-gations contributing to a patient's diagnosis, only a few are suitable for the diagnosis of cancer. However, asymptomatic patients with cancer can have higher levels than symptomatic patients. The markers may provide information about the patient's prognosis, enabling the appropriate therapy to be used. A tumour marker may be used as a non-invasive method to measure the patient's response to treatment, once the initial baseline has been established.

Clinicians may overlook requesting a tumour marker test at the pre-treatment stage. Although the results may not contribute to the diagnosis, it is essential to establish a pre-treatment baseline sample if the tumour marker is to be used to monitor the patient's response to treatment. Decrease in the marker level may be an indication that the cancer has responded favourably to therapy. In cases after surgery or radiotherapy, this would suggest that treatment has been successful. Conversely, if levels remain constant, or indeed rise, it may be an indication that the tumour is not responding to treatment, signalling recurrence or progression of the tumour (Bidart et al., 1999). A rise in a tumour maker's level may be used as an early warning sign and may precede confirmation of the presence of a tumour by imaging investigations by up to several months.

However, once a patient's tumour markers are measured by one laboratory, the same laboratory should be used for testing all subsequent serial/longitudinal samples from the patient to maintain consistency, i.e. the same assay methodology is used. Different values may be obtained between laboratories, even for those using automated systems, as seen from analysis of results from external quality control assurance schemes (Sturgeon and Seth, 1996; Sturgeon et al., 1999a, 1999b). Table 8.1 lists tumour marker-associated tumour sites.

Table 8.1 Examples of some of the most frequently requested tumour markers and their associated cancers

Tumour marker	Associated tumour
a_1-Fetoprotein (AFP)	Liver, germ cell (testis, ovary)
β_2-Microglobulin (β_2M)	B-cell lymphoma, multiple myeloma, chronic lymphocytic leukaemia
β Human chorionic gonadotrophin (β-hCG)	Choriocarcinoma
Cancer antigen 15-3 (CA15-3) or BR27.29	Metastatic breast cancer
Carbohydrate antigen 19-9 (CA19-9)	Pancreatic and colon cancer
Cancer antigen 125 (CA125)	Epithelial ovarian cancer
Carcinoembryonic antigen (CEA)	Gastrointestinal tract cancer; breast; liver and lung
Cytokeratins	Transitional cell carcinoma
Lactic acid dehydrogenase (LDH) isoenzyme 5	Germ-cell tumours
Neuron-specific enolase (NSE)	Neuroblastoma, pancreatic small cell lung carcinoma
Prostate-specific antigen (PSA)	Prostate cancer
Prostatic acid phosphate (PAP)	Prostate cancer
Thyroglobulin	Thyroid cancer
Vanillylmandelic acid (VMA)	Neuroendocrine tumours

Laboratory aspects

Assay technology

Tumour markers are predominately measured by immunochemistry techniques (IHC, fluorescence *in situ* hybridization (FISH) and immunoassays). There are a number of different assay formats used, depending on the technology platform employed. Most immuno-assays for tumour markers use the two-site immunometric (sand-wich) immunoassay format, depending on the available epitopes present on the antigen concerned. The assay format often employs a matched pair of monoclonal antibodies, or a monoclonal and a poly-clonal antibody specific for the marker concerned. One is used as a capture antibody bound to the solid phase, whereas the other is used as a labelled detection antibody. The sample from the patient is incu-bated in the captured antibody solid phase, and any specific antigen in the sample is then bound to the antibody, with unbound material being removed by washing. The detection antibody is added, which binds to any captured antigen. Unbound detection antibody is removed by washing and the bound detection antibody is measured. An alternative to the sequential assay approach is a simultaneous immunometric immunoassay format, where the detection antibody can be incubated at the same time as the patient's sample.

Another format often used is the competitive immunoassay, e.g. in the case of CA27.29, where there is a single epitope, recombinant CA27.29 antigen is bound to the solid phase. The sample from the patient is then incubated in the solid phase in the presence of labelled detection antibody. Antigen in the patient's sample competes with the antigen bound on the solid phase for the labelled antibody. Any detection antibody that has bound to the antigen in the sample, and not to the solid-phase antigen, is removed by wash-ing. The presence of labelled detection antibody is then measured. Reduction in the labelled detection antibody signal is an indication that the detection antibody has bound to the antigen in the patient's sample. Absence of antigen in the patient's sample would be indi-cated by high detection antibody signal, i.e. detection of antibody binding to the antigen on the solid phase.

A number of different technologies are used in employing differ-ent detection systems. For ^{125}I-radiolabelled antibody (radioim-munoassay or RIA) a gamma counter is used to measure the gamma emissions; for colorimetric enzyme system (enzyme-linked immunosorbent assay – ELISA or EIA), the absorbance of the colour change of precipitating substrate in the presence of the enzyme labelled antibody is measured spectrometrically; for luminescence systems light-emitting substrates are measured in the presence of enzyme-labelled antibody either by luminometer or using enhanced luminescence with time-resolved imaging and a charged coupled device (CCD) camera; for fluorescence, using fluorescein- or fluorophore-labelled antibody, emission of fluorescence at specific wavelengths is detected by photodetector/CDD camera after excitation at another wavelength by polarized light or a laser. Figure 8.1 shows a sandwich assay.

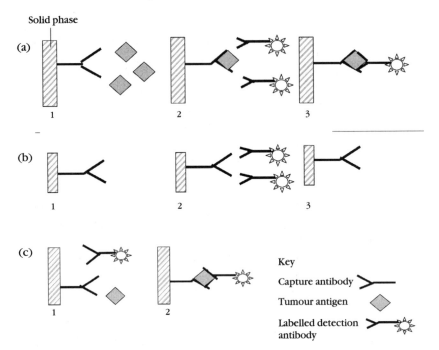

Figure 8.1 Immunometric sandwich assay. The various stages of two sandwich assay formats are shown: (a) sequential and (c) simultaneous. In (a): 1, sample incubated on the solid phase coated with capture antibody for a specific tumour antigen; 2, after washing to remove any unbound antigen, labelled detection antibody for specific antigen is added to the solid phase and incubated; and 3, after washing any labelled detection antibody that has bound to antigen/capture, antibody complex is then detected. (b) The results of an unreactive sample, absence of antigen/capture antibody/labelled detection antibody complex.

Quality assurance and standardization

Quality assurance is fundamental for any diagnostic laboratory test for performance and reporting of the assay results. Awareness of the limitations of the assay should avoid any adverse effect on patient treatment.

One of the problems with tumour marker assays has, in the past, been the lack of standardization, i.e. one assay may not be comparable to another for a particular marker. One antibody derived against a particular antigen can have a different affinity and specificity for an epitope from another, and it may recognize only a subunit of the antigen rather than the total antigen.

The International Society for Oncodevelopmental Biology and Medicine (ISOBM) is addressing this issue by validating and characterizing the antibodies, and mapping the epitopes to which the antibody is raised. The monoclonal antibodies against a particular tumour marker are compared and assessed for their suitability as 'capture' or 'detection' antibodies, and how they perform as a matched pair. This evaluation is usually conducted by comparison of the performance of different manufactured assays for a particular assay. The ISOBM has also agreed on the structure of some of the marker antigens (Nustad et al., 1996; Stenman et al., 1999).

These assays now have to meet more stringent regulation requirements on their suitability for diagnostic use, i.e. validation and reproducibility data, worldwide. In the USA, only a few tumour marker assays have received approval by the Food and Drug Administration (FDA), e.g. CA27.29 and CA125. In Europe, the In Vitro Diagnostic Directive (IVDD – Directive 98/79/EC) is addressing the problem of comparability between kits. Kit standards are required to be referred to and to correspond to available international reference standards for each tumour marker. A number of manufacturers with assays using similar formats are already collaborating in the calibration of their kit standards to this specification. The use of tumour marker reference control sera in these assays is strongly recommended to assist standardization between laboratories and manufacturers' kits (Sturgeon and Seth, 1996; Sturgeon et al., 1999a, 1999b; Sturgeon, 2001)

To date, many tumour markers still lack an agreed international reference standard. Another problem is the lack of agreed consensus about reference ranges for tumour markers. These can vary by tenfold or more. In general, users of the same methodology quote similar ranges. The guidelines from the Association of Clinical Biochemists in Ireland (1999) recommend that reference ranges should be used only for guidance and trends in changes of levels are more clinically useful than absolute values. Laboratory reports should reflect this.

The participation in external quality control assessments (proficiency) is helping to standardize tumour marker testing between laboratories, e.g. an EORTC external quality programme for ER and progesterone receptor (PgR) measurement between 1998 and 1999 has been examining the two different assays used, a ligand-binding assay (LBA) and an EIA in 42 and 39 participants, respectively. The initial results showed the coefficient of variation (CV) between laboratories for the two assays to be 40–50%. After normalization of the results, CV values between laboratories dropped to 11% for ER LBA and 14% for ER EIA. The results demonstrated the need to calibrate assays between laboratories, an essential requirement to enable the use of data obtained in multicentre clinical studies (Sweep and Geurts-Moespot, 2000).

The 1999 consensus recommendations of the European Group for Tumor Markers (EGTM) are that performance CVs for most tumour markers assays on automated systems of < 5% (intra-assay) and < 10% (interassay) are achievable.

In addition, the testing laboratory must ensure good laboratory practice (written protocols for validated assays, frequent equipment calibration, assay run acceptance criteria and monitoring, i.e. Westgard rules, documentation audit trials, etc.).

One of the most essential procedures should be the use of internal quality control (IQC) samples in every assay, which should fall within the detectable range for that assay. The IQC sample must mimic the patient's samples and must not be from the same manufacturer of the assay, i.e. independent of the assay manufacturer. The use of IQC samples ensures that the assay is robust and reproducible and, used with the Westgard rules, it will highlight any system failure, e.g. requirement for recalibration (Westgard et al., 1981; Westgard and Barry, 1986). The laboratories performing these investigations should be accredited and able to demonstrate their quality system by audit to external peer reviewers.

Understanding the limitation of an assay used for a tumour is essential to avoid erroneous results. One such aspect is sample collection intervals for monitoring a patient, which is related to the kinetics of serum tumour marker concentrations. Knowledge of the tumour marker half-life or doubling times is important when scheduling sampling time between samples. Bidart and his colleagues (1999) suggested that:

> . . . the use of tumour kinetics rather than cut-off values may often provide the most relevant predictive factors for the estimation of disease-free and overall survival, treatment efficacy, and for the decision regarding optimal treatment and cost-effectiveness in terms of toxicity and patient benefit . . .

Limiting factors, such as interference in assays from auto- and heterophilic antibodies in the patient's sample leading to erroneous results, are well known (Kricka, 2000; Marks, 2002).

The use of monoclonal antibody therapy has now led to another possible source of interference, i.e. human anti-mouse monoclonal antibodies (HAMAs). In the USA, the FDA requires that the assay manufacturers specifically draw attention to HAMAs as a potential problem. It is essential that the clinician provide all the relevant clinical information when requesting a tumour marker test, in particular that any monoclonal therapy received by a patient is clearly indicated. The laboratory can then perform appropriate pre-treatment to the sample before it is tested for a tumour marker (Marks, 2002).

Another problem can be an inappropriate sample type. In the case of VEGF measurements, citrated, EDTA-treated or heparinized plasma in glass containers is the sample of choice. If serum samples are used, VEGF can be released from platelets and other blood components during blood clotting, leading to increased levels compared with plasma samples (Webb et al., 1998; Adams et al., 2000). (It is advisable to refer to your local pathology laboratory's testing schedule for the service that they offer and their sample requirements for a particular test.)

What is the usefulness of tumour markers in disease management?

The decision to test for tumour markers can depend ultimately on a clinician's management for a patient. To provide patient care, several guidelines have now been produced by a number of expert panels. Examples include guidelines by the ASCO. It recommends that only oestrogen receptor and progesterone receptor values are of benefit in predicting which breast cancer patients are suitable for endocrine therapy (ASCO, 1996, 1998; Hammond and Taube, 2002). The College of American Pathologists (CAP) has evaluated tumour markers, in both 1994 and 1999, and has identified those that it recommends for clinical use for breast, prostate and colon cancer (Henson et al., 1995; Hammond et al., 2000; Hammond and Taube, 2002).

The reviews of the various guidelines from multidisciplinary expert panels at international, national and regional levels have found that, although substantial research has been or is being performed in the field of tumour markers, very little has been done on how this translates into clinical practice (Hayes et al., 1998; Sturgeon, 2002).

Fleisher and his colleagues (2002) have comprehensively reviewed these expert panel guidelines. They were based on stringent methodologies for preparing clinical practice guidelines, and are regularly reviewed and updated to reflect evidence-based publications. In most cases the evidence-based references were cited.

Sturgeon, one of the authors of the Fleisher review, has written a further outline summary of their work (Sturgeon, 2002). Sturgeon found that the guidelines could be categorized into two groups: (1) tumour markers for specific cancers (ASCO) and (2) tumour markers for a range of cancers (EGTM, ABCI, NACB). Their recommendations were fairly general, providing advice about which markers to measure in specific malignancies and their appropriate application. The guidelines were found to focus either on clinical aspects (surgery, etc.) or on laboratory investigations. Overall the guidelines provided valuable consensus documents on the management of specific cancers; they should be referred to when drawing up local protocols. A multidisciplinary team approach, consisting of both the clinicians and the laboratory scientists, should be taken when drawing up local protocols (DoH, 2000b). Sturgeon suggested that consideration should be given to how best to implement, publish, disseminate and promote ownership of the local protocol. She recommended the development of audit procedures to monitor the effectiveness to clinical practice.

Useful markers for disease management

The guidelines agreed, with the exception of prostate cancer, that tumour markers, (primarily as a result of specificity and sensitivity) should not be used for screening. Otherwise, they are involved in staging and prognosis, detection of recurrence, follow-up and monitoring.

The most common serum tumour markers used as surrogates, to monitor the course of disease during and after treatment, in clinical use are: CA-125 for ovarian cancer, CA19-9 for ovarian cancer, CEA for colorectal cancer, prostate-specific antigen (PSA) for prostate cancer, and AFP and β-human chorionic gonadotrophin (β-hCG) together with the isoenzyme lactic acid dehydrogenase (LDH) for germ-cell tumours.

As a result of low sensitivity and low specificity of CA15-3, or BR27.29, it is not recommended that these MUC-1 tumour markers are used for screening, diagnosis or staging of breast cancer. However, they can be useful in determining metastatic disease (Molina et al., 1999; Bast et al., 2001).

Prostate-specific antigen (PSA) is another controversial marker as a result of the false-positive and false-negative results when used as a screening test. When used for screening in men aged over 50 years, or those at high risk (family history of prostate cancer), it is necessary to include a digital rectal examination as part of the screening assessment (Lamerz et al., 1999; Semjonow et al., 1999; American Urological Association, 2000).

The future role of tumour markers in disease management

Since 1997 there has been major funding by the National Cancer Institute (NCI) in the USA on research for new diagnostic, prognostic and predictive cancer markers. Funding is also provided for translating research techniques that have been used on cell lines or animal models into clinical use, to assist oncologists when selecting the correct treatment strategies.

Completion of the first stage of the Human Genome Project has provided sequence data and has advanced to the next stage of confirming the gene sequence, as well as identifying the expressed products of these genes (Collins et al., 1998).

The NCI has established the Cancer Genome Anatomy Project (CGAP), which is developing a catalogue of genes associated with cancer. This resource for reading the molecular signatures/portraits of cancer from mRNA-extracted material of archived paraffin-embedded tissue is compared with normal tissue using analysis of gene chips to find those with increased or decreased expression of specific mRNAs (Strausberg et al., 1997, 2000). To date, over 1 000 000 gene expressed sequence tags (EST) have been deposited in this public bioinformatics cDNA library database, together with their histological reports, TNM (tumour, node, metastasis), staging and clinical outcome data (Lal et al., 1999; Strausberg, 2001; Strausberg et al., 2003).

Work is now under way to identify proteins associated with the expressed mRNA using proteomics. Outcomes of this research are expected over the next 10 years. One of the main aims is to identify suitable early detection cancer tumour markers and other markers for predicting prognosis. The results of ongoing clinical studies, using existing tumour markers, may provide information on which are the best to use (NCI, 2001).

The next few years will see a further development in assay technology, 'protein chips'. These chips will include miniaturized versions of existing tumour assays, allowing multiplex testing on small sample volumes using high-throughput systems, contributing to a tumour profiling approach for patients with cancer.

Other approaches are being investigated to examine circulating autoantibodies which are raised against the tumour markers themselves. In patients with cancer, these would be expected to be higher than in cancer-'free' individuals. In the case of MUC-1, serial serum samples from primary breast cancer patients showed significant correlation between tissue staining and circulating autoantibodies.

As a result of the heterogeneous nature of cancers the use of multiple biomarkers can increase the sensitivity of tumour markers (Cheung et al., 2002).

The appropriate use of tumour markers will greatly assist the clinical management of an individual's cancer in the future. Such 'tests' will aid the monitoring of a patient and potentially alert the clinician at an earlier stage to a possible recurrence, thereby influencing survival.

CHAPTER 9

Monoclonal antibodies

HELMOUT MODJTAHEDI

Background

Cancer is the leading cause of death in developed countries. Despite major advances in chemotherapy, treatment of cancer patients with cytotoxic drugs, in particular those with metastatic solid tumours, does not induce complete remission in the great majority of patients. As cytotoxic drugs are not specific for tumour cells, there is often a wide range of toxicity associated with the use of such drugs in patients and the development of drug resistance phenotypes is a major cause of treatment failure. Therefore, identification of antigens that play an important role in tumour pathogenesis and specific targeting of such antigens with a new generation of specific anti-cancer drugs is essential if we are to win the battle against cancer. Indeed, since the 1900s, one major goal of scientists is the ability to produce large amounts of a single type of antibody against a tumour antigen that could then be used as a 'magic bullet' in the treatment of cancer (Dillman, 1989; Ward et al., 1997; Gura, 2002).

In 1975, Köhler and Milstein developed a procedure called hybridoma technology for the production of monoclonal antibodies in mice. This technology, which allows the production of unlimited quantities of a specific type of antibody (monoclonal antibody or mAb) against any target antigen, has revolutionized many areas of biological and medical research. As a result of the specificity of an mAb for a particular antigen, mAbs have been generated against a wide range of antigens in the past 28 years. Monoclonal antibodies have become essential tools in our understanding of the function of many genes and their protein products; in the discovery of novel tumour antigens and for the diagnosis of cancers and in tumour classification. In addition, as a result of recent advances in genetic engineering, and our better understanding of cancer biology, tumour antigens and tumour immunology, monoclonal antibodies are now being used for the treatment of cancer patients (Waldman, 2003).

109

Since 1986, 11 monoclonal antibodies have been approved by the US Food and Drug Administration (FDA) for the management of a wide range of human diseases including the prevention of graft rejection and treatment of autoimmune disease and cancer (Gura, 2002). Of these, three unconjugated mAbs have been approved for the treatment of human cancers. In other instances, mAbs have been conjugated to other therapeutic agents such as radioisotopes or drugs in order to increase the specific delivery of such agents to tumour cells. Currently, mAbs account for about 30% of all new biotechnology drugs in development, with more than 400 at different stages of clinical trials worldwide.

In this chapter, the structure and function of mAbs (naked and conjugated) are discussed, together with the principle of this therapeutic approach. Recent advances in mAb technology and our understanding of tumour antigens, which have ultimately led to the current use of mAbs in the management of human cancers, are also covered. In particular, there is a focus on a number of mAbs such as trastuzumab (Herceptin) and Rituxan, which are currently used in the treatment of metastatic breast cancer and haematological malignancies, together with some discussion of newer mAbs (e.g. anti-human epidermal growth factor receptor mAb), which are likely to be approved for the treatment of cancer in the near future.

What are antibodies and monoclonal antibodies?

Antibodies are immunoglobulins (Igs) that are produced after the exposure of activated B lymphocytes to a particular antigen (Figure 9.1). They are Y-shaped structures which are present on the surface of B lymphocytes or circulate in the bloodstream after secretion by a differentiated form of B lymphocytes called plasma cells. All antibodies have the same basic structure and consist of two identical heavy (H) chains and two identical light (L) chains which are held together by disulphide bonds (Figure 9.1). Both heavy chains and light chains are further divided into variable (V) or constant (C) regions. The variable portion of both the heavy and light chains (V_H and V_L) forms the two identical antigen-binding fragments (Fab) of the antibody. The constant portions of heavy chains, called crystallizable fragment (Fc), are responsible for the activation of the complement system and alerting the host immune system to attack the target antigen (Figure 9.1a).

One of the useful characteristics of antibodies is that they are extremely specific for a particular antigen. Until 1975, it was not possible to produce large amounts of an antibody directed against a

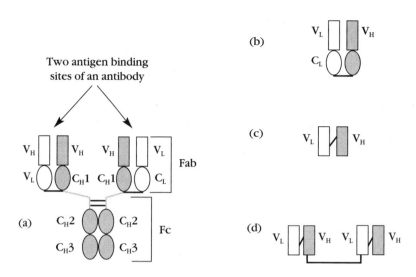

Figure 9.1 Structure of an intact antibody (immunoglobulin) and antibody fragment developed by genetic engineering for tumour imaging and therapeutic applications. An intact antibody consists of two identical heavy chains and two
identical light chains connected by disulphide (-S-S-) bonds (a). Both heavy
(larger) chains and light (smaller) chains contain a constant portion (C_H and C_L
respectively) and a variable portion (V_H and V_L respectively). The antigen-binding
site of an antibody is located at the variable domain of the antibody (i.e. V_H and V_L)
and the antibody's immunological effect is mediated by the constant (Fc) portion
of an antibody. To increase tumour penetration, smaller fragments of antibodies,
such as monovalent Fab, scFv or divalent $(scFv)_2$, have been generated which
retain the antigen-binding specificity of intact antibody. (a) Intact divalent IgG
molecule (150 kDa; (b) monovalent Fab (55 kDa); (c) monovalent scFv (30
kDa); and (d) divalent $(scFv)_2$ (60 kDa).

specific antigen (Köhler and Milstein, 1975). Before 1975, antibodies
were generated by the immunization of a group of animals with a
particular antigen (e.g. viruses, bacteria, tumour cells) on several
occasions. Then sera were collected from such animals and used for
the treatment of patients who had the same infection. Unfortunately,
the administration of the crude preparation of sera from immunized
animals, which also contained other animal proteins, produced
strong allergic reactions in many such patients. In addition, when a
recipient animal (e.g. a sheep, a rabbit or a mouse) is immunized
with an antigen, serum from such animals contains a mixture of
different antibodies. These antibodies, which are produced by different populations of B lymphocytes, are called polyclonal antibodies.
Sera from such immunized animals may therefore contain very low
levels of therapeutic antibodies, which, for example, could block
the binding of infectious agents to human tissues and cause their

eradication by activating the patient's immune system. Furthermore, as a result of the short survival of B lymphocytes from immunized animals in culture, the large-scale production of antibodies from a single clone of B lymphocytes was not possible until the innovation of the hybridoma technology by Köhler and Milstein in 1975. Using this technology, the antibody-producing B lymphocytes from the spleen of immunized animals were immortalized by the fusion of their cell membrane with a continuous proliferation of myeloma cells, in order to produce a single antibody-secreting cell called a hybridoma (Köhler and Milstein, 1975). The procedure for the production of monoclonal antibodies by hybridoma technology is shown in Table 9.1.

Table 9.1. Production of monoclonal antibodies by hybridoma technology

1. Immunization of animals (mouse or rats) with antigen X.
2. Removal of B lymphocytes from the spleens of immunized animals.
3. Immortalization of antibody-producing B lymphocytes by fusion of their cell membrane with myeloma cells (i.e. hybridoma production).
4. Growth of hybridoma cells in a 96-well plate containing special cell culture medium.
5. Screening of hybridoma supernatants for antibodies to antigen X.
6. Cloning of hybridomas that secrete anti-X antibodies by limiting dilution (i.e. by adding a single hybridoma per well of the tissue culture plate).
7. Growth of the hybridoma cell in culture so that they become confluent.
8. Re-testing of the hybridoma supernatant for antibodies against antigen X.
9. The positive hybridomas are re-cloned once more, expanded in culture and some are frozen in liquid nitrogen for later use.
10. Once required, hybridoma cells secreting a single type of antibody against antigen-X (i.e. monoclonal antibody) are grown in culture medium and the antibodies secreted into the culture medium are purified for therapeutic and/or diagnostic purposes.

Using hybridoma technology, mAbs have been prepared against a wide range of antigens, including growth factors, growth factor receptors, tumour-specific antigens, viruses, bacterial products, hormones, drugs, enzymes and differentiated antigens. Such antibodies are used routinely in the identification of such antigens in human tumour biopsies and sera, and in investigating their role in tumour progression. Köhler and Milstein were awarded the Nobel Prize for Medicine in 1984, as a consequence of the great impact of hybridoma technology on medical sciences.

Engineered antibodies

These include chimeric antibodies, humanized antibodies, human antibodies and antibody fragments. As described above, the first panel of monoclonal antibodies was developed against human tumour antigens in mice (Köhler and Milstein, 1975). Although mouse antibodies are very useful as diagnostic agents and in the unravelling of the biological and clinical significance of human tumour antigens, their therapeutic application in patients may be limited because of their immunogenicity (Dillman, 1989; Coghlan, 1991). When repeated doses of antibodies from a non-human source (e.g. mouse antibodies) are given to patients, such antibodies may be recognized as 'foreign' by the patient's immune system and lead to the generation of a human anti-mouse antibody (HAMA) response. This in turn may lead to the rapid elimination of the administered antibody from the patient's bloodstream before producing therapeutic effects (Ward et al., 1997).

Chimeric and humanized antibodies

With advances in genetic engineering in the 1980s and 1990s, the immunogenicity of mouse antibodies has been reduced by several methods (Hudson and Souriau, 1993). In some instances, the chimeric format of mouse antibodies has been developed by transferring the antigen-binding domain (V_H and V_L) of mouse antibody into a human IgG framework (Figure 9.2). Chimeric antibodies, which are a 30% and 70% mixture of mouse and human sequences respectively, are expected to be less immunogenic than mouse antibodies (see 'Rituxan' below). Humanized versions of mouse antibodies have also been developed by transferring three stretches of amino acids in the variable region of mouse antibodies (CDRs), which are responsible for the binding to the antigen, into the human IgG framework (Figure 9.2). The resultant humanized antibodies contain more human sequences (90%) and should be less immunogenic than rodents and chimeric antibodies in cancer patients (see 'Herceptin' below). Most clinical trials currently under way, together with those approved for the treatment of cancer patients, are using the chimeric or humanized form of mouse antibodies (Hudson and Souriau, 1993) (Table 9.2).

Human monoclonal antibodies

Since the early 1990s and as a result of further advances in molecular biology, it has become possible to develop fully human mAbs against human tumour antigens (Winter and Milstein, 1991; Marks and Marks, 1996; Glover, 1999; Davies et al., 1999). The two techniques

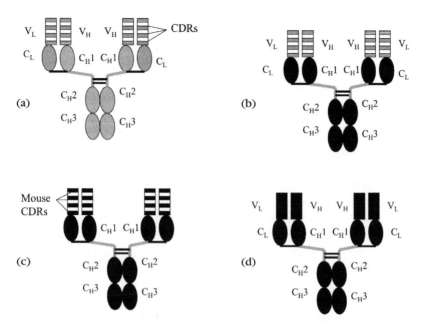

Figure 9.2 Structure of (a) mouse (first generation, 1970s), (b) chimeric (second generation, 1980s) and (c, d) humanized (third generation, 1990s) monoclonal antibodies developed for therapeutic applications. The chimeric monoclonal antibodies contain 66% human sequence and 34% mouse (V_H and V_L) sequence and are generated by the fusion of DNA from the mouse variable region to DNA from a constant region of human IgG antibody. In contrast, humanized antibodies contain more than 90% of human sequences and are formed by fusion of DNA for three stretches of amino acids from the mouse variable domain into a human IgG framework.

used for the development of human antibodies against human antigens are the phage display technology and the use of transgenic mice, XenoMouse animals. In the latter case, the mouse antibody gene has been replaced by a human antibody gene. The immunization of such transgenic mice with human tumour antigens has led to the development of human antibodies in such animals. Clinical trials with a number of fully human mAbs are currently under way worldwide (Yang et al., 2001). The results should indicate whether chronic (i.e. repeated) treatment of cancer patients with human mAbs is less immunogenic than chimeric antibodies and humanized mAbs, which are directed against the same tumour antigen.

Antibody fragments

Preclinical and clinical studies with radiolabelled antibodies have indicated that intact antibodies such as whole IgG (160 kDa) are too large for rapid penetration of solid tumours and have slow blood

Table 9.2 Monoclonal antibodies that have been approved by the US Food and Drug Administration for cancer therapy

Antibody	Target antigen	Antibody format	Disease	Year approved
Rituximab (Rituxan)	CD20	Chimeric	Non-Hodgkin's lymphoma	1997
Trastuzumab (Herceptin)	HER-2	Humanized	Breast cancer	1998
Gemtuzumab ozogamicin (Mylotarg)	CD33	Humanized (attached to toxin)	Acute myeloid leukaemia	2000
Alemzutumab (Campath 1H)	CD52	Humanized	Chronic lymphocytic leukaemia	2001
Ibritumomab tiuxetan (Zevalin)	CD20	Mouse (attached to radionuclide)	Non-Hodgkin's lymphoma	2002

clearance. With the advances in genetic engineering, smaller fragments of the antibodies such as Fab (55 kDa) and scFv (30 kDa) have been developed to retain a single antigen-binding fragment (i.e. monovalent) of the intact divalent antibody (see Figure 9.1b–d). Smaller fragments of such antibodies can be attached to radioisotopes for in vivo imaging or therapy of tumours, because they can penetrate tissue more effectively and clear faster from a patient's peripheral circulation (Hudson and Souriau, 1993).

The mechanism of action of monoclonal antibodies

As each antibody is highly specific for a particular antigen, this characteristic feature of the antibodies has led to their widespread use in diagnostic kits, basic research and more recently cancer management. In addition, after the recent success in mapping of the human genome, mAb technology has become an essential tool in the discovery of novel human tumour antigens that are overexpressed in human malignancies and in the identification of antigens, which are differentially expressed between the primary and metastatic tumours (Holt et al., 2000).

Depending on the subclass (Fc portion) of antibodies and the antigens recognized by such antibodies, mAbs can produce their anti-tumour activities by several mechanisms, see Table 9.3.

Monoclonal antibodies can inhibit the growth of tumours by blocking the binding of growth factors, which are essential for

Table 9.3 Mechanisms by which monoclonal antibodies produce therapeutic effects

- Unconjugated monoclonal antibodies (i.e. unmodified):
  - by blocking the binding of growth factors to their receptors, which is essential for tumour proliferation
  - by inducing programmed cell death (i.e. apoptosis)
  - by binding to effector cells (e.g. natural killer or NK cells) and inducing antibody-dependent cellular cytotoxicity (ADCC) at the tumour sites
  - by activating complement and inducing complement-dependent cytotoxicity (CDC).

- Conjugated monoclonal antibodies: by attachment to the following agents a lethal dose of such molecules can be delivered to tumour cell:
  - toxins (e.g. diphtheria toxin, pseudomonas exotoxin)
  - radioisotope (e.g. iodine-131, yttrium-90)
  - bispecific mAbs (e.g. MDX-210) enhance tumour destruction by host effector function.

tumour cell proliferation, to such receptors, e.g. the human epidermal growth factor receptor (EGFR) is a 170-kDa transmembrane cell surface glycoprotein that transmits the mitogenic action of the EGF family of growth factors, such as EGF, transforming growth factor α (TGFα), HB-EGF (heparin binding-epidermal growth factor), BTC (betacellulin) and epiregulin. From histological examination of human tumour biopsies, it has become evident that overexpression of EGFR, accompanied by co-production of one or more of its ligands, is a common feature of human tumours of epithelial origin (Modjtahedi and Dean, 1994). Overexpression of EGFR has been detected in cancer of the bladder, breast, lung, brain, stomach, prostate, ovary, pancreas, and head and neck. This in turn has been associated with a poor prognosis in many such patients (Modjtahedi and Dean, 1994; Nicholson et al., 2001).

In recent years, several laboratories have generated a panel of mAbs against the external domain of EGFR, which blocks the binding of the ligands to EGFR and inhibits the growth in vitro and in vivo of a wide range of human tumours that overexpress EGFR. On the basis of these studies, a panel of anti-human EGFR mAbs (e.g. IMC-C225 (chimeric antibody), ICR62 (rat) ABX-EGF (human antibody), EMD 777 (humanized antibody)) is currently at different stages of clinical trials in a wide range of cancer patients, either alone or in combination with chemotherapy or radiotherapy (Modjtahedi et al., 1996; Mendelsohn, 2001; Yang et al., 2001; Needle, 2002).

Monoclonal antibodies may also induce anti-tumour activity in vivo by directing ADCC and mediating CDC (Ward et al., 1997) (see Chapter 6). These effector functions of the antibodies are dependent on the Fc portion (i.e. subclass) of antibodies, e.g. human IgG1 antibodies are ideal for inducing ADCC at the tumour sites by binding to human mononuclear NK cells and macrophages. When a human IgG1 antibody binds to a target antigen on the tumour cell surface, via their Fab domain, the Fc portion of such antibodies can also bind to Fc receptors on circulating NK cells and macrophages. The binding of such immune cells to antibodies at the tumour sites can mediate ADCC in such target cells. The results of preclinical studies with a panel of mAbs have shown that the anti-tumour activity of mAbs improves substantially in vivo, when such antibodies could also trigger ADCC by bringing cytotoxic T lymphocytes, NK cells and other immune effector cells to the tumour sites (Berger et al., 2002).

As explained above, each antibody molecule has two identical antigen-binding domains. To enhance the effector function of an antibody, bispecific mAbs have been generated that are directed against two different target antigens, with one arm binding to the tumour antigen and the other to the antigen on host immune cells (e.g. CD3 antigen on T cells). A number of phase 2/3 clinical trials with different bispecific mAbs are currently under way in several clinics worldwide. The results of such trials should unravel the full potential of this new approach in cancer therapy (Cao and Lam, 2003).

In other cases, mAbs have been attached to cytotoxic drugs, radioisotopes or enzymes in order to deliver the lethal doses of such molecules to tumour cells and in tumour imaging (Pagliargo et al., 1998; Dillman, 2002; Fracasso et al., 2002; Yao et al., 2002). However, ideally in such cases the antigen should be overexpressed on malignant tumours with no, or a very low level of, expression in normal tissues. The characteristics of ideal antigens as targets for mAb-based therapy are given below.

- Overexpression of target antigens on tumour cell surfaces.
- No or limited level of expression of antigens on normal cell surfaces.
- Homogeneous expression of antigens on tumour cells.
- No shedding of tumour antigens in patients' sera, which can trap the administered therapeutic antibody progression.

Monoclonal antibodies that are currently used in cancer therapy

There are currently five mAbs commercially available, which have been approved for the treatment of haematological cancers and breast cancer (see Table 9.1). The characteristic features of these antibodies, together with the antigens recognized by them, are discussed below.

Rituxan antibody (rituximab)

Rituxan was the first monoclonal antibody that was approved by the US FDA for the treatment of cancer in 1997. Rituxan is a chimeric mAb (34% mouse protein and 66% human protein) and is directed against B-lymphocyte-restricted differentiation antigen CD20. It has been developed by transferring the entire Fab domain of mouse anti-CD20 antibody to the human IgG1 framework (Hainsworth, 2000).

CD-20 antigen is expressed on the surface of more than 90% of B-cell non-Hodgkin's lymphomas (NHLs), on pre-B lymphocytes and on mature lymphocytes, but not on stem cells, plasma cells and other normal tissues. B-cell lymphoma accounts for 95% of all lymphomas.

Rituxan is jointly marketed by two American companies (IDEC Pharmaceutical and Genentech, California) for short-course outpatient treatment of relapsed or refractory CD20-positive, low-grade or follicular B-cell NHL. Rituxan is a less toxic alternative to chemotherapy and can induce anti-cancer activity by binding to CD20-positive cells, inducing apoptosis, recruiting immune effector functions (i.e. mediating ADCC) and activating complement (Scott, 1998; Hainsworth, 2000). As a single agent, rituximab has been shown to produce a response rate of 50% in patients with relapsed low-grade and follicular NHL. When added to standard chemotherapy in patients with diffuse, large, B-cell NHL, it has also been able to prolong survival in such patients (Dearden, 2002). Treatment-related toxicity, which occurs most often with the first infusion of the antibody, is generally mild. Infusion-related reactions included rigors, nausea, urticaria, fatigue and headache (Dillman, 2002). One advantage of Rituxan therapy is that, as it induces minimal adverse effects, it can be given to patients as short-course, outpatient therapy (375 mg/m^2 weekly for 4–8 weeks). Further clinical trials examining the clinical benefits of adding Rituxan to conventional chemotherapy, using different schedules, are currently under way (Dearden, 2002; Foran, 2002).

The mAbs epratuzumab and apolizumab, which are directed against two different antigens CD22 and HLD-DR respectively, are also under clinical investigation for use in NHL (Leonard and Link, 2002). Simultaneous targeting of CD20, CD22 and HLA-DR antigens in patients with NHL by antibodies may produce a better therapeutic benefit in such patients, compared with those who are treated with one antibody. Further clinical trials in patients with NHL, with a combination of Rituxan, epratuzumab and apolizumab, should unravel the full potential of such strategies.

Herceptin (trastuzumab)

Herceptin was the first therapeutic monoclonal antibody that was approved by the US FDA for the treatment of solid tumours in 1998 (Bell, 2002; Freebairn et al., 2001). Unlike Rituxan, Herceptin is a humanized antibody, which is directed against the external domain of the human epidermal growth factor receptor-2 (HER-2). It has been approved for the treatment of patients with metastatic breast cancer whose tumours overexpress HER-2 receptors.

HER-2 is a non-mutated, tumour-associated, cell surface antigen and a member of the type I growth factor receptor family (Rubin and Yarden, 2001). Overexpression of HER-2 has been shown in 20–30% of patients with breast cancer and in a number of other epithelial tumours (Walker, 2000). In addition, high levels of expression of HER-2 have often been associated with more aggressive disease, poor response to the conventional form of therapy, increased risk of metastasis and poor survival in patients with breast cancer (Cook et al., 2001). As HER-2 overexpression plays an important role in the clinical behaviour of human tumours and is responsible for a poor response to conventional forms of therapy, such antigens form an ideal target for mAb-based therapy (Green et al., 2000; Rubin and Yarden, 2001).

In the past 15 years, a panel of mouse and rat mAbs have been generated against the external domain of HER-2 for both diagnostic and therapeutic applications in oncology (Sliwkowski et al., 1999; Baselga and Albanell, 2001). HER-2 blockade by mAbs has been shown to inhibit the proliferation of the HER-2 overexpressing tumours both in vitro and in animal models (Baselga and Albanell, 2001). Of the anti-HER-2 antibodies studied, the mouse anti-HER-2 mAb 4D5, which showed potent anti-tumour activity and specificity in preclinical studies, was selected for humanization, by the American Biotech Company Genentech (Carter et al., 1992). The humanized form of mouse anti-HER-2 mAb 4D5 (i.e. Herceptin) was generated by transferring the CDR from mAb 4D5 into a human IgG1 framework (Carter et al., 1992). Preclinical studies with Herceptin have shown that it can induce anti-tumour activity against HER-2-overexpressing tumours by several mechanisms, including downregulation of HER-2 from the cell surface and its subsequent mitogenic signal, cell-cycle arrest, induction of apoptosis, inhibition of angiogenesis, activation of complement and mediation of ADCC at tumour sites by binding to effector cells such as NK cells (Sliwkowski et al., 1999; Harries and Smith, 2002). In addition, Herceptin has been shown to increase the anti-tumour activity of cytotoxic drugs against HER-2-overexpressing human breast tumour cell lines in preclinical settings (Baselga et al., 1998; Baselga and Abanell, 2001; Sliwkowski et al., 1999).

Clinical trials with Herceptin in breast cancer patients, both as single agent and in combination with cytotoxic drugs such as paclitaxel, have shown that it improves survival in such patients (Harries and Smith, 2002). In particular, the benefit of therapy with Herceptin was more evident in patients whose tumours expressed the highest level of HER-2 (3+). The results of clinical studies have also indicated that, although Herceptin is well tolerated in the great majority of such patients, cardiac toxicity is seen in a minority of patients (about 2%) treated with Herceptin alone. This was greater in patients who received Herceptin in combination with an anthracycline regimen (26–28%). Further studies, using Herceptin in combination with a newer generation of cytotoxic drugs and/or other biological agents, are currently under way which could in turn lead to the development of more effective therapeutic regimens for these highly aggressive, HER-2-overexpressing, metastatic breast cancers (Bell, 2002; Ligibel and Winer, 2002). In addition, recent studies have indicated that some cancer patients, whose tumours are HER-2 positive, may also shed some HER-2 antigen into their sera (Hait, 2001). Such shed antigens in turn may trap some of the administered Herceptin, thereby reducing the effective dose reaching tumour sites. In such cases the dose of Herceptin administered to patients should be increased to compensate for the antibodies trapped by shed antigens.

Campath 1 (alemtuzumab)

Alemtuzumab is a humanized mAb that is directed against the CD52 antigen (Waldman, 2003). The CD52 antigen is present on the surface of normal T lymphocytes, B lymphocytes and a high proportion of lymphoid cancers, but absent on haematopoietic stem cells. The original rat monoclonal antibody against CD52 was generated in Cambridge, in the UK, in 1980 and the humanized version of this antibody was approved by the FDA for the treatment of chronic lymphocytic leukaemia (CLL) in 2001. This antibody is able to 'kill' CD52-positive target cells by activating complement and by mediating ADCC (Dearden, 2002; Waldman, 2002). It induces remission in about a third of patients with fludarabine-refractory B-CLL (Foran, 2002). Recent studies suggest that alemtuzumab may be most effective in patients with minimal residual disease or when used in combination with cytotoxic drugs such as fludarabine (Dearden, 2002). However, this antibody induces immunosuppression, as a result of depletion of normal B and T lymphocytes, causing an increased risk of opportunistic infections in such patients (Pangalis et al., 2001; Rai et al., 2002).

Conjugated monoclonal antibodies in cancer therapy

As explained above, in some cases mAbs have been attached to modified toxins or radioisotopes in order to deliver lethal doses of such molecules to tumour cells. Ideal antigens for such therapeutic strategies are tumour-specific antigens. Two conjugated mAbs that have been approved for the treatment of human cancers are described here.

Immunotoxin: Mylotarg (gemtuzumab ozogamicin)

Mylotarg is the first toxin-linked antibody that has been approved for the treatment of human cancer. It is a humanized anti-CD33 mAb which is attached to the cytotoxic anti-tumour antibiotic, calicheamicin

(Berger et al., 2002). It has been approved by the US FDA, as a single agent for the treatment of patients with CD33-positive acute myeloid leukaemia (AML) in the first relapse who are over the age of 60 and not suitable for therapy with conventional cytotoxic drugs (Berger et al., 2002; Dearden, 2002). AML is the most common type of acute leukaemia in adults and is characterized by accumulation and proliferation of myeloblasts in the bone marrow.

The CD33 antigen is not expressed on stem cells or non-haematopoietic normal cells but has been shown to be expressed on myeloblasts in 80–90% of patients with AML. The binding of this immunotoxin to CD33 antigen on AML cells results in the internalization of the immunotoxin and dissociation of calicheamicin; its transport into the nucleus and the degradation of the DNA lead ultimately to cell death. Clinical studies with Mylotarg, as a single agent in patients with CD33-positive AML, produced a complete response rate of 15–20% (Berger et al., 2002).

Radiolabelled mAbs as radioimmunoconjugate agents

The goal of radioimmunotherapy (RIT) is to deliver cytotoxic radiation from therapeutic radioisotopes to tumours using mAbs (similar to a guided missile) that bind to those cells expressing the target antigen (Hainsworth, 2000; Cheson, 2001). The success of RIT depends on several factors, including the choice of the target antigens, antibody molecules (guided missiles) and therapeutic radioisotopes (Juweid, 2002), e.g. ideally the target antigen should be tumour specific and expressed only on tumour cells with no level of expression on normal cells. In practice, most of the target antigens recognized by antibodies are tumour-associated antigens that are also present in lower numbers on the surface of normal cells. To minimize exposure of such normal cells to the radioisotope, a relatively high dose of unlabelled antibody is given to the patients, either before or with the administration of various radiolabelled antibodies. The two most common isotopes that are used in RIT are iodine-131 (^{131}I) and yttrium-90 (^{90}Y) (Dillman, 2002; Juweid, 2002). The advantage of radioimmunotherapy over unconjugated antibodies in cancer therapy is that the former has a longer path, which allows further deeper penetration and killing of tumour cells (both antigen positive and negative) without direct binding of antibody to such tumours.

Ibritumomab tiuxetan (Zevalin) is the first RIT agent that was approved for the treatment of cancer in February 2002 (Dillman, 2002). Zevalin is a ^{90}Y-labelled anti-CD20 antibody (IDEC Pharmaceuticals, USA) which has been shown to produce a 74% response rate in Rituxan-refractory NHL patients. To determine the relative efficacy of

Zevalin (^{90}Y-labelled anti-CD20 antibody) to unconjugated anti-CD20 antibody (Rituxan) in the treatment of patients with NHL, 143 NHL patients were randomized into two groups, in a phase 3 clinical trial. The overall response rate in patients treated with Zevalin and Rituxan was 80% and 56% respectively. As explained above, the advantage of RIT over unconjugated mAb is that the former penetrates deeper into the tumour mass and can also kill antigen-negative tumours in a crossfire effect. Therefore, patients who are not responsive to, or relapse after chemotherapy or treatment with unconjugated antibodies, may be suitable candidates for RIT approaches (Dillman, 2002; Foran, 2002; Juweid, 2002).

Future considerations

Since the discovery of hybridoma technology, mAbs have been generated against a wide range of human tumour antigens. These antibodies were subsequently used to unravel the importance of such antigens in the biology of cancer, as diagnostic agents, and more recently in cancer treatment. Unfortunately, the first generation of mAbs that were generated in mice were immunogenic in cancer patients. This in turn prevented repeated administration of such antibodies, limiting their efficacy. After advances in genetic engineering, it has become possible to develop the recombinant form of mice monoclonal antibodies (i.e. chimeric or humanized). Three such unconjugated antibodies are currently being used in the management of cancer patients, because such antibodies prolong survival. More importantly, patients treated with mAbs do not develop high-grade side effects which are often associated with the use of conventional chemotherapy. In other cases, the anti-tumour activity of mAbs has been enhanced by conjugating to toxins and radioisotopes, in order to deliver lethal doses of such molecules to tumour cells. Although antibodies such as Rituxan and Herceptin are very useful in the treatment of cancer patients, the duration of response in some patients may be short (less than a year). Therefore, with the identification of other cell surface antigens of biological and clinical importance, and by simultaneous targeting of such antigens with mAbs and other therapeutic strategies, it should be possible to prolong survival in most cancer patients. Indeed, the results of ongoing clinical trials of hundreds of mAbs, which are directed against a wide range of human antigens, should unravel their full potential as 'magic bullets' in the treatment of human cancer.

PART III
FROM RESEARCH TO
TREATMENT

CHAPTER 10

What is translational oncology?

ELAINE VICKERS

'Is it something to do with genetics?' 'Is it about converting some-thing into something else?' 'Haven't got a clue.' In fact all three are correct. Translational oncology or translational research is a new term without any real consensus about its meaning. The *Concise Oxford English Dictionary* (Allen, 1990) describes translation as:

> the process of moving something from one place to another.

Indeed, many have similarly described translational oncology as 'bench to treatment couch'.

When thinking of cancer research, be it prevention, diagnosis or treatment, one tends to think of two areas: the laboratory-based researchers – workers in white coats and pipettes who inject test tubes or culture Petri dishes – and clinical trials where patients are directly involved in the testing of a substance or treatment. Transla-tional oncology aims to bring the two dimensions together and make the laboratory work relevant to clinical practice.

What exactly is translational oncology?

Researchers in basic biomedical science strive to unravel the work-ings of a physiological process. They want to understand how things do or do not work in many cases. This is important and ground-breaking work, but many patients and health professionals could argue 'so what, if it doesn't improve clinical outcomes?' The informa-tion learnt will no doubt contribute to the enormous knowledge and evidence base and help in the understanding of individuals, but will it really impact on better cancer treatments?

Translational research attempts to bridge the gap between test tube and patient, to ensure that the new scientific findings are translated into new developments, either diagnostically or therapeutically.

Importantly the fundamental purpose of the research is improved clinical practice. Translational research takes something from the scientific arena to a patient and brings back questions from the patient to the scientists. This is not as easy as it sounds. Scientists do not always regularly read medical journals and medics do not generally read scienctific journals. Blagosklomy (2002) agrees with this statement and urges that data published in scientific journals be translated into detailed treatment protocols which can be directly used by a doctor and tested in a clinical trial. His thoughts are not unique. Birmingham (2002) quotes Professor Nadler who states:

> I can't train the next generation because there is now an enormous amount of science and no one to bring it to patients.

What translational oncology is not

Many think that they are translational oncologists or involved in translational research, but many are misguided. Those involved in the following are *not* examples of translational researchers:

- cloning genes from a human cell line or tissue
- studying human specimen profiles on chips
- developing new classes of drugs
- company-based phase 1 trials.

Those who *are* translational researchers are, through their own work, attempting to:

- improve diagnosis for patients
- improve the prognosis for patients
- improve cancer prevention
- conceive or execute new treatment.

(Birmingham, 2002)

Looking at the lists above there is potential benefit in bringing the knowledge of the researchers in the first list together with that of the researchers in the second list.

How will bringing the sciences together be achieved?

Searching the internet and libraries for examples of translational oncology research reveals not only individual examples of 'bench-to-treatment couch' research but entire programmes of research, including a coordinated approach to the subject in the UK. The

National Translational Cancer Research Network (NTRAC) has been established to speed up the processes by which laboratory-based research becomes a therapeutic treatment that will benefit cancer patients. NTRAC currently incorporates eight centres of scientific and clinical research, each being selected by the Department of Health and cancer stakeholders. The centres are currently: Birmingham, Leeds, Newcastle, Southampton, the Royal Marsden, Imperial College London and University College London, with the possibility of Cambridge, the Manchester and other centres joining shortly. This network is funded by the Department of Health and has an overall aim to increase:

- the number of new treatments and diagnostic tests
- the number of early clinical trials
- the number of patients across the country taking part in these trials.

(www.ntrac.org.uk)

As well as this coordinated approach, many other centres exist in isolation that do equally valuable work. Their fundamental aim is to develop laboratory work into new therapies and in so doing improve outcomes for patients.

Before looking at specific examples of translational oncology, it is worthwhile looking at the breadth of translational work. The following is taken from NTRAC (2002).

Within the remit of translational research areas of work can include the following:

- Small molecules: research has provided considerable insight into the molecules and pathways involved in transforming a normal cell into a cancer cell (see Chapter 4). These *changes* are being examined by scientists in striving to develop drugs that will inhibit or regulate their abnormal activity. Cancer Research UK is leading the development of novel anti-cancer agent treatments emerging from cancer research.
- Gene therapy and cancer vaccines: viruses can be genetically modified to carry a tumour-specific antigen. These are currently being developed for a range of cancers. This work will test the hypothesis underpinning vaccine development and included in it are mechanistic biological endpoints such as virus distribution, immunological evidence or induction of T-cell response (see Chapter 7).
- Novel diagnostics: new and improved technologies developed from the genome knowledge are helping in the search for novel

diagnostic, prognostic and predictive factors. These techniques will help the clinician to subdefine disease and tailor therapy to the individual patient, i.e. select anti-cancer therapies on an individual basis rather than a population basis. Projects of this type require close collaboration between those scientists who developed the technology and the clinicians who manage specific cancers (see Chapter 8).

• Hypothesis testing in clinical communities: this could involve assembling national DNA or cancer tissue banks. This will enable the clinical community to search for genes, proteins or other molecules that contribute to the clinical behaviour of different cancers.

These examples are cited as being dynamic processes that depend on the fusion of expertise. The bench researcher fully integrates with the front-line clinician and vice versa. To bring the start of this chapter alive and demonstrate translational oncology in practice, it is useful to work through a couple of areas of research.

Angiogenesis

Angiogenesis is one example of laboratory research translated into clinical practice. It is the growth of a new blood supply from pre-existing vasculature. The existing capillaries sprout new branches to serve and nurture the tumour. This is triggered by proteins known as tumour angiogenesis factor and involves numerous biological activities (Tortora and Grabowski, 2003).

Preclinical studies have demonstrated the major role of angiogenesis, tumour growth and formation of metastases, which lead to the thinking that suppression of the blood supply suppresses the tumour (Pinedo and Salmon, 2000). Most cancer treatments have been targeted at killing the cell. Although treatments have been modified and refined over the past 50 years, the aim of treatment remains targeted at the same tumour cell. An understanding of angiogenesis and the notion that the tumour is angiogenesis or blood supply dependent have led to the second target in cancer treatment – the newly formed capillaries.

As mentioned above, the current thinking is that cancer treatment targets the cancer cell to cause cell death. Folkman et al. (2001) suggest that the cancer genome is clever in its make-up, continually mutating or changing at both primary (main) and distant (secondary or metastases) sites. This creates challenges for the clinical staff because eventually these changes will create a resistance to the drugs targeted at them. In stark contrast, the cells that line the new capillaries at the tumour site are stable with a virtually non-existent mutation or change rate. These cells, known as microvasculature endothelial cells, are needed for further tumour growth which makes them a very powerful player in any malignant process. These endothelial cells not only supply oxygen and nutrients to the tumour; it is now known that they also provide a gateway for anti-apoptotic factors, or anti-switch-off factors, and so protect the tumour by allowing its cells to go into mass production. Simply, what the above is saying is that we know that a tumour continually changes its make-up and that it is dependent on a blood supply. The ever-changing nature of the tumour cells may result in drug resistance. Added to this, the blood supply remains constant, supplying nutrients so that the tumour thrives.

Killing the blood supply will kill the tumour whether or not mutated and drug resistant. This is the basis of *this* translational research.

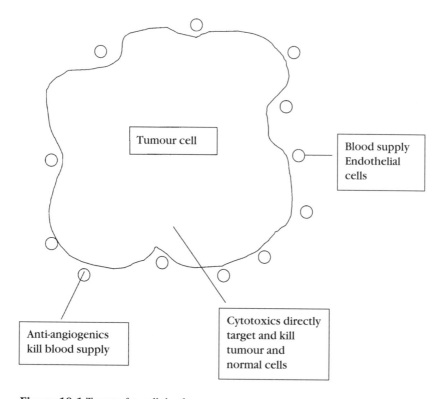

Figure 10.1 Targets for cell death.

Preclinical and clinical work is ongoing. Some centres use anti-angiogenesis agents alone and/or in combination with chemotherapy. The aim is to inhibit tumour growth, reduce metastases, prolong survival and improve quality of life (Pinedo and Salmon, 2000). However, is it possible to have concurrent use of cytotoxic chemotherapy and anti-angiogenic agents? If the blood supply is suppressed, how do the cytotoxic drugs reach the tumour? This is a valid concern, but one that has not yet been elucidated. Animal studies of lung cancer by Leicher, cited by Pinedo and Salmon (2000), demonstrated a synergistic effect. Combination therapy reduced not only the number of metastases but also the size of the metastases, providing evidence that anti-angiogenic therapies can improve treatment.

How is knowledge about angiogenesis changing practice?

Angiogenesis inhibitors

The cells that line the newly formed capillaries (microvasculature endothelial cells) supply the nutrients that encourage the tumour to thrive. Angiogenesis inhibitors are a new class of drug that work specifically to inhibit proliferating and migrating endothelial cells. Many of these drugs have now reached phase 3 trials. These drugs work in two ways and are summarized in Table 10.1.

Currently there is no test or assay to determine the best approach/dose in an individual patient. The challenge for scientific researchers is to develop a simple test to measure the effect of angiogenesis inhibitors, which will aid clinicians in refining treatments to individual needs.

It is hoped that, from this example, the role that scientists play in the quest to improve the outcome for the patient can be demonstrated: true 'bench to treatment couch' oncology research.

Table 10.1 Anti-angiogenesis: mode of action

	Direct action	Indirect action
Target cell	Endothelial cell	Tumour cell
Effect	Prolonged use as a result of little or no drug resistance	Resistance possible caused by tumour cell mutation
Example	Endostatin	Herceptin

Imatinib mesylate

Another example of translational oncology/research is one of the great successes of recent years, and this is the story of imatinib mesylate (Glivec) has dramatically changed the lives of patients with chronic myeloid leukaemia (CML). CML is a disease of the myeloid stem cell characterized by marked splenomegaly and an increase in the production of white cells. The natural course of CML is a chronic phase, as described above, moving into an accelerated or blast crisis that, untreated, leads to death in a matter of weeks. Treatment aims at controlling the white blood cell count with splenectomy and the chemotherapy drugs busulphan, hydroxurea or interferon. These measures can control the disease for a number of years. Bone marrow transplantation provides the only chance of cure, but only 20% of CML patients are eligible for this highly toxic treatment. Since the development and clinical use of imatinib mesylate, treatment approaches have changed. Traditional chemotherapy aimed at killing the mutant cancer cells; bone marrow transplantation cured 'by replacing the blood making cells'; now imatinib mesylate targets and blocks the *cause* of CML.

Where did it all begin?

The story began 40 years ago in the 1960s. Researchers in Philadelphia were able to identify a common genetic mutation in patients with CML. Chromosome 22 had a 'bit' missing. This became known as the Philadelphia chromosome and was found in 95% of CML patients, and was the first time that a genetic abnormality had been linked to a specific cancer. It took a further 13 years to find the 'missing bit'. It had moved to chromosome 9. This phenomenon of moving from one chromosome to another is known as 'translocation'. The Philadelphia chromosome was now known as a translocation from chromosome 22 to chromosome 9. This was the first time that this phenomenon had been observed. Since then, many other translocations have been detected

The next chapter of the CML story was the identification by the scientists of a rogue enzyme produced by the Philadelphia chromosome known as Bcr-Abl. This enzyme changes the cell's activity and causes the cell to go into mass production, the characteristic of CML. The high white cell count seen in a peripheral blood count is a result of this enzyme switching on the mass production button. Scientists knew the genetic mutation for CML and had identified the single enzyme that switches on mass production. This left a clear direction for laboratory research to have an impact on the patient outcome and to demonstrate true translational oncology, namely:

Block Bcr-Abl → Block overproduction → Control/cure disease

This challenge was taken up and in 1995 scientists had developed a potent specific inhibitor of Bcr-Abl. Preclinical work was encouraging and in the laboratory the inhibitor (now known as imatinib) did not demonstrate significant activity against normal cells, in stark contrast to traditional chemotherapy treatment. Clinical trials began and, in 1998, 31 patients were entered into a trial using imatinib. All 31 had a complete haematological response to treatment and one-third had a cytogenetic response, i.e. elimination of the Philadelphia chromosome. After these exceptional results phase 2 trials were initiated and produced the same exciting results. In addition, imatinib was well tolerated and had very few side effects. Again the improved patient outcomes were a direct result of the collaboration of laboratory scientists and clinical staff, not forgetting the pioneering and brave patients.

The continued success of imatinib in the treatment of CML is one of the major breakthroughs in cancer care over the past decade. However, the story, although dramatic, is incomplete. Imatinib resistance has now occurred in some patients and a dermatological side effect has emerged. This clearly defines the next step for the scientists to find out why!

Angiogenesis and the imatinib story, although different, are clear examples of scientists and clinicians working together with the same aim – better patient outcome.

What of the future?

The coordinated approach now being taken to translational research/oncology shows the commitment from both the laboratory and clinical fields to improving outcomes. This can only be of huge benefit to patients, but is the NHS ready for their findings?

- Can the NHS cope with individualized treatments for patients?
- Can expertise be sustained?
- Can the multidisciplinary teams cope with the time and effort involved in individualizing treatment en masse?
- Are the hospital-based laboratories equipped for new technology?
- Can the health economy sustain new treatments?
- Are there any savings for the health economy from improved outcomes?
- Will there be any delay in starting treatment while refining the individual plan?
- Are patients willing to wait for treatment?

These are real issues the NHS must face. Translational oncology research offers a fantastic opportunity to get research and clinical experts working together to improve outcomes for patients but at a financial cost. Time will tell if we as a society can afford the price tag.

CHAPTER 11

The application of research methodology to cancer research

CARMEL SHEPPARD

> Unfortunately the impressive list of advancements in the science of medicine appears to have led to a decline in the art of medicine. Patients complain increasingly that 'high tech' medicine dehumanises them. In the eternal quest for a new and better treatment for every known ailment we have started to forget the other important needs of sick people
>
> Fallowfield (1990, p. 16)

The preceding chapters of this book have focused principally on the 'scientific' advances in cancer treatment that have been primarily led by scientists and consequently mostly lie within the biomedical domain. This never-ending search for a greater understanding of what causes cancer, the biological effect of cancer on the body, and the search for new drug regimens to improve survival or even cure cancer are essential and give hope to us all. Indeed the recent improvements in cancer survival rates demonstrate the advances made through such clinical research. Many patients' lives have been extended and enhanced through the introduction of new treatment regimens. Nevertheless, it is important not to forget the individual in all of this, who has to cope with the consequences of treatment, live with the knowledge of a life-threatening illness and the devastating psychological effects that this brings to the patient and family. In the past decade it has been encouraging to see this aspect of care incorporated into many national clinical trials and the growing recognition of its importance. This is illustrated by the emergence of quality of life as a required endpoint of many trials. However, although some progress has been made overall, there remains a paucity of nursing research to support certain nursing interventions, e.g. the advantages of specialist nursing intervention, as well as evidence relating to survivorship and rehabilitation, and the relationship between nursing and patient outcomes (Corner, 2002; Richardson et al., 2002). Following a literature review between 1980 and 2000, only

446 articles pertaining to cancer nursing research were identified, with less than 50% of these reporting primary nursing research (Richardson et al., 2002).

Why do we need to continue to develop a research-based knowledge in cancer nursing? Research is the means through which we can gain a deeper understanding of the effects of cancer, formulate questions about patient care, test the effectiveness of pre-existing treatment and care, and in turn generate new ideas and evidence for practice. Understanding the effects of cancer and its physical and psychological impact will inevitably enable nursing to prepare patients more readily and support patients experiencing similar circumstances. Ultimately, through research we aim to improve the overall quality of care for patients. In addition, through nursing research we can strengthen the ability and opportunities for nurses to influence health-care policy by identifying the priorities and requirements of the future health service (DoH, 2000c). Sadly, the ability to do this has been hampered by the lack of research-based knowledge from which to draw, in comparison to our medical colleagues. It is not therefore surprising that health-care policy has been traditionally dominated by medicine. To ensure that patients benefit from a truly multidisciplinary approach to care, it is essential that we strive to develop this knowledge base. To do so is dependent not only on time and funding, but also on the ability to produce well-designed research that generates meaningful results. Richardson et al. (2002, p. 7) suggest that 'nursing research has too often been hampered by a limited focus, small sample sizes or inadequate rigour'. Although nurse education now includes training in research methodology, this has not always been the case, and the general prevailing culture in nursing outside academic institutions does not appear to sustain a major commitment to research. Richardson et al. (2002) identified that less than half (44%) of lead cancer nurses identified current nursing research initiatives in their clinical areas.

The Department of Health document *The Nursing Contribution to Cancer Care* (DoH, 2000d) suggests that one of the main barriers to research is the lack of training in this area. One of the functions of this chapter is to provide the reader with a basic understanding of research design, setting out steps towards developing a research proposal, as well as being a useful guide to critiquing published research.

Research is sometimes viewed as a series of complex methodological investigations reserved for academics, yet as nurses we are frequently engaged in research without realizing it. Research questions should be formulated within clinical practice, e.g. where there is limited evidence to support a particular aspect of clinical care, or through the observation of certain trends while working with a group of patients, or concerns relating to treatments. Some clinical areas have developed journal clubs that serve as a vehicle through which debate can be encouraged and ideas generated for investigation.

A well-structured proposal is a prerequisite for any research investigation. This should follow a systematic set of rules, which importantly demonstrate that rigour has been applied to the study. A research proposal should include a literature review that justifies the need for research in a given area. The overall aims and objectives of the project should be stated and, if the project aims to test theory (deduction), the hypothesis should be stated. The design of the study, the sample unit, methods of data collection and analysis should be presented and justified. In developing a study several considerations should be made:

- What is the topic to be investigated? This should be clear, focused on a specific aspect, free of ambiguity and achievable.
- What sort of information is needed before the start of the research, i.e. literature search, anecdotal evidence?
- What sort of evidence is needed to answer the question?
- What type of investigation would provide the evidence needed?
- What are the resources required for the study, e.g. time, finances, supervision etc?
- What is a realistic time frame for the study?
- How will the results be disseminated?

The design of the study should be that which answers the question best. In reality the design is often determined not only by the question but also by the philosophical underlying assumptions/ perspectives of the researcher, which fall into either positivist or naturalistic perspectives, sometimes referred to as quantitative or qualitative research, respectively. Costs, time and expertise will also to some extent influence the design the study.

Quantitative research

Biomedical research is dominated by quantitative research drawing from the positivist paradigm (Black, 1994); the underlying philosophical principles are that all human behaviour occurs through external stimuli, which can be observed and measured. The way in which the phenomenon is measured is usually through quantitative research, which begins via the generation of ideas about the phenomenon of interest and subsequently develops ways to support or reject the hypothesis created. This form of research is particularly useful in gaining information about the effectiveness of treatment and patient outcomes in response to treatment in terms of generalized numerical data, and hence differs from the qualitative approach, which focuses on the subjective experiences of individuals.

Sample sizes should be stated in the proposal. In quantitative research sample size is generally calculated at the outset of the study and this is essential if the researcher wishes to have a high chance of detecting any statistically significant effect. It is advisable to seek advice from a statistician who can assist in the calculation of sample size. The researcher attempts to demonstrate that the difference between any two groups relates to the treatment or what is being tested, and nothing else. As we can never be absolutely sure that what is observed relates only to what is being tested, the significance level (p value) is generally set at between 0.01 and 0.05 and is determined by the researcher (i.e. a 1–5% chance that the differences were not caused by the hypothesis). This level of significance is the degree of risk that the researcher is willing to take that they reject the null hypothesis when it is really true, otherwise known as a type I error. A type II error is when the researcher mistakenly accepts a false null hypothesis. Samples that are too small have a high risk of failing to demonstrate a real difference. Some academic journals now decline publication of data from small studies unless other sources of information published in the related field are limited. Importantly, if statistical power is low the results of the study may be heavily criticized – 'statistical power is a measure of how likely the study is to produce a statistically significant result for a difference between groups of a given magnitude (i.e. the ability to detect a true difference)' (Bowling, 1997, p. 149). It is normally accepted that the power of a study should be between 80 and 90% (i.e. you have an 80–90% chance of detecting a statistically significant result) (Bowling, 1997; Salkind, 2000; Greenhalgh, 2001).

A further consideration is the sampling methods to avoid unwanted bias and to ensure that the sample is representative of the particular patients under investigation. There are basically two types of sampling to include: probability and non-probability sampling; however, in quantitative research the main aim of the study is to ensure representation of the target population, so probability sampling is the preferred method. There are a variety of approaches to probability sampling to include simple random sampling, systematic random sampling, stratified random sampling and cluster sampling, which are described further by Bowling (1997) (Table 11.1).

Table 11.1 Randomization sampling frame

Simple random sampling	Each participant has an equal chance of being selected for either the control or the experimental group
Stratified random sampling	If the sampling frame contains a large variation in variables, i.e. age, disease site, etc., the researcher may wish to ensure that the sample is representative. According to the variables, units are separated in the sample frame into strata (layers) and samples are drawn from each stratum
Cluster sampling	Units are divided into groups that are subsequently sampled randomly (usually used for economic purposes). Again there may be difficulties with clusters being unrepresentative, e.g. involving participants from a shared environment may not be truly reflective of the total population
Systematic sampling	Units are selected at intervals from lists, i.e. every fifth patient on the list. The researcher should be aware, however, of the potential bias that lists may have

When designing the study the researcher must consider the tools of measurement that can be varied, e.g. patient satisfaction may be measured by postal questionnaire, structured and semi-structured interviews or telephone interviews. Justification of the methods used should be stated in the proposal. Issues such as cost and increasing the opportunity for greater response rates and convenience for the patient will usually influence the decision concerning how data will be collected. If a questionnaire is used, care should be taken in the design to ensure that participants can clearly understand what is requested of them, that it is presented in such a manner so as to encourage completion and that it is free from ambiguity, all of which may affect the ability later to analyse the results. Issues of confidentiality should also be considered so that participant answers are not influenced by the possibility of being identified. A pilot study should be undertaken to test the questionnaire before the final study to confirm that the questions measure what they are intended to measure before large-scale implementation. One of the increasing areas of investigations is patient-based outcomes. Measurements of quality of life, psychological morbidity and attitudes tend to be complex and any measurement tool should be tested for both reliability and validity. Reliability is the extent to which the instrument demonstrates reproducibility and consistency through repeated administration (Bowling, 1997). 'Validity is an assessment of whether an instrument measures what it aims to measure' (Bowling, 1997,

p. 130). Numerous tools have already been developed and tested, e.g. the General Health Questionnaire (Goldberg and Williams, 1988) and the Hospital Anxiety and Depression Scale (Zigmond and Snaith, 1983), both of which measure psychological morbidity. Quality-of-life tools are also available (Bowling, 2001), some of which have been specifically designed for studies relating to cancer, such as the Functional Assessment of Cancer Therapy (Cella et al., 1993) and the EORTC Quality of Life Questionnaire (Sprangers et al., 1993). Other measurements may include clinical outcome measures, e.g. numbers of tumours detected or recurrence of tumour, which may be collected either retrospectively or prospectively from the patients' medical/nursing notes, or service outcomes and cost-effectiveness.

Generally quantitative research produces large quantities of numerical data that are presented either in descriptive form (data that describe the characteristics of a sample or population) or as inferential statistics (data that enable inferences from the sample data to be applied to a population) (Salkind, 2000). How the results are to be analysed and presented should be considered in the proposal and design of the study.

Although there is a variety of approaches to quantitative research, three main designs are described below, although these should not be viewed as exhaustive of quantitative designs.

Randomized controlled trials

The randomized controlled trial (RCT) is generally referred to as the gold standard of research and is often used to compare interventions. It is basically an experimental trial comparing two or more groups who are randomly allocated to either one form of treatment or another. It is through this random allocation that the risk of extraneous variables is reduced, thus increasing the chance that any changes are caused only by the intervention, so allowing the cause and effect to be determined. The essential characteristics of this design include a hypothesis that one form of treatment or intervention will cause a particular effect (e.g. the nurse may develop a hypothesis that wound healing is improved with the use of a particular dressing and he or she may then aim to test this hypothesis). Second, the study is prospective in nature and patients are randomly allocated to receive either the intervention (i.e. the dressing to be tested) or the control (which in this case would be the accepted standard form of dressing). The researcher attempts to eradicate bias through the randomization process, thus comparing two groups who are very similar, apart from the variable under investigation (e.g. the dressing) (Figure 11.1).

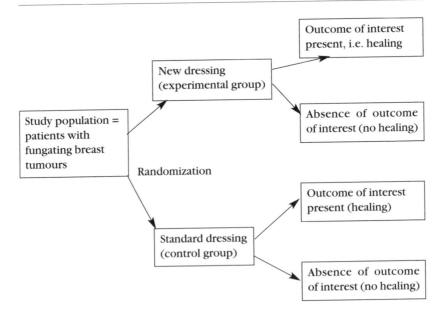

Figure 11.1 Basic design structure for randomized controlled trials (RCTs).

As well as investigating the effects of certain types of interventions, drugs or procedures, the RCT is also useful in determining the most appropriate provision of care. RCTs are not appropriate for studies where there is difficulty in randomization, e.g. it would be unethical to randomize patients into certain arms of treatment where one particular treatment is known to have superiority. There are also some variations of RCT design, an example of which is the simple crossover method. This allows both groups to act as their own control by exposing them sequentially to both arms of the study. However, this would not be suitable for conditions that fluctuate before treatment, and also if there were residual effects of the first arm of the treatment causing potential bias (Bowling, 1997)

Example: RCT used in cancer care (Baildam et al., 2001)

Objective

To compare nurse-led versus doctor-led follow-up after a diagnosis of breast cancer and completion of treatment.

Design

After a diagnosis of breast cancer, patients are generally followed up by their consultant or registrar for a period of 5–10 years. This randomized study compared follow-up by two specially trained experienced specialist nurses (experimental group) versus the traditional follow-up with doctors (control group).

Sample size

In total 525 patients were randomized to each of the groups.

Outcome measures

This included differences in detection of recurrence between the two groups, recognition of patient psychological morbidity and patient satisfaction between the two groups. Psychological morbidity was measured using well-validated measurement tools to include the Hospital Anxiety and Depression Scale (HAD) and the Spielberger State Anxiety. Satisfaction was also measured using the Fallowfield Satisfaction with Consultation Questionnaire.

Results

The results demonstrated that nurse recognition of psychological morbidity was greater than that recorded by the doctor. No differences in the ability to detect recurrence were found. The authors conclude that nurse-led clinics can provide high-quality care equal, at least, to that of their medical colleagues.

Quasi-experiments: case–control studies and cohort studies

A case–control study may be used to investigate a problem related to a cause of disease. Patients with a particular condition (cases) are compared with an identical group of individuals who do not have the condition (controls). Both groups should be identically matched except for the condition under study. Case–control studies are generally retrospective, and accounts of past history and exposure are investigated to ascertain the common lifetime exposures, linking these to possible causation of disease. The benefits of this form of research are that the researcher can study multiple exposures and diseases that have long latent periods, e.g. breast cancer may recur some 15–20 years later, hence the benefits of breast screening should be evaluated over this time. It is also useful in situations where it would be unethical to carry out an experimental study and where little is known about the cause of the disease. The evidence gained from this sort of research generally is considered lower down the ladder of hierarchical research compared with the RCT. There is potential to overlook influencing factors that may have been outside the realms of the study, and thus the results may be less reliable. There may also be difficulties with selection bias, particularly as the researcher must attempt to rule out other possible threats to the validity of the findings, i.e. other exposures. Information bias may also be a potential problem because exposure status is determined after the outcome has occurred and therefore participants' recall of exposure may be blurred.

Example of case–control (Draper et al., 1997)

Objective

To test the hypothesis that 'childhood leukaemia and non-Hodgkin's lymphoma can be caused by fathers' exposure to ionising radiation before the conception of the child, and more generally, to investigate whether such radiation exposure of either patient is a cause of childhood cancer'.

Design

The case group (35 949 children diagnosed with cancer) were compared with the control group (a group of individuals selected from the birth register for the same area of birth, matched on sex and born within 6 months of the case).

Outcome measures

These included (a) parental employment as radiation worker before conception of child, (b) cumulative dose of external ionizing radiation for various of periods of employment before conception of child, and (c) dose during pregnancy.

Results

Although the researchers confirmed that the fathers of the children with leukaemia or non-Hodgkin's lymphoma were significantly more likely than fathers of controls to have been radiation workers, they concluded that this did not relate to a preconceived radiation dose. As such the absence of a relationship between dose and risk led the researchers to believe that these findings may be related to either chance or perhaps some characteristic other than exposure to radiation.

Cohort studies

Cohort studies can be prospective or retrospective (historical), depending on the time that the exposure data were measured. The essential feature of all cohort studies is that the exposure is measured before outcome (Greenhalgh, 2001). In a prospective cohort study, the researcher begins with individuals who have not yet had the outcome of interest (e.g. bowel cancer) and follow the group forward in time measuring exposure (e.g. exposure of interest may be diet) to see if the outcome of interest occurs (i.e. bowel cancer diagnosis). In a retrospective cohort study exposure is measured using data collected before the study started (i.e. looking back through case notes at the main exposures during the study period), although recall bias may be an issue with retrospective data. In addition to bias, Brennan and Croft (1994) highlight the importance of confounding which must be considered in any cohort study. Unlike the RCT, in which participants are randomly allocated to either the experimental or the control arm, participants of cohort studies have chosen to be exposed or not and subsequently this in itself may affect the outcomes of both groups. 'As a consequence, if a confounder is not recognised and adjustments made for its effect the exposed and unexposed groups in such studies will not be comparable' (Brennan and Croft, 1994). Figure 11.2 shows a cohort study design.

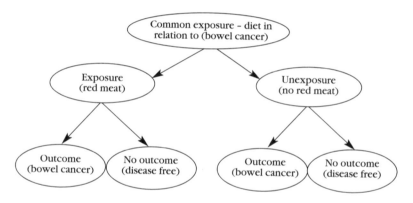

Figure 11.2 Cohort study design.

Example of a cohort study (Graham et al., 2002)

Objective

To confirm the relationship between severely stressful life experiences and relapse of breast cancer found in a previous case–control study.

Design

This was a prospective study recruiting a cohort of women newly diagnosed with breast cancer. The researchers controlled the group for a biological prognostic factor (i.e. other factors that might affect recurrence rates such as lymph node status and tumour grade).

Outcome measure

Recurrence of disease.

Data collection

Women were interviewed every 18 months over a period of 5 years, collecting data on stressful experiences and depression (including data on experiences 12 months before diagnosis).

Results

Overall the researchers found no increased risk of recurrence in women who had one or more severely stressful life experiences in the year before diagnosis compared with women who did not, and of those who had stressful experiences since diagnosis the results demonstrated a lower risk of recurrence, hence confirming that stressful events did not lead to increased risk of recurrence.

The interesting thing about this study is that it is a good example of how different designs may affect research outcome. As the researchers themselves point out, their findings differ from those in an earlier study (Ramirez et al., 1989) which used case-controlled methods. The researchers suggest that this may relate to difficulties, in retrospective studies, in recalling stressful experiences and the possibility that patients look back for something to blame for the development of recurrence, so a prospective study enables greater recall and accuracy of data.

Descriptive and analytic surveys

Descriptive surveys are designed to measure a particular phenomenon within a cross-section of the population, e.g. in cancer care this design may be used to identify the prevalence of cervical cancer in the Jewish population, or perhaps the prevalence of cervical cancer in women who have had numerous sexual partners. Consequently, surveys are retrospective and can be used to generate a hypothesis, or test hypothesis, e.g. cervical cancer is more common among women with multiple sexual relationships. The benefits are that large numbers of people can be surveyed, although, as with any retrospective data, recall may add bias. In addition surveys cannot be used to indicate a direction of cause.

Analytic surveys are longitudinal and record data at frequent intervals, making this approach useful in monitoring the effects of interventions, e.g. health promotion activities, through observation of changes in lifestyle patterns. One of the difficulties is the possibility of sample attrition, and the prospective approach means that results can take time, and tend to be expensive particularly in relation to administration costs. Furthermore, in both these designs survey information tends to be superficial, and breadth rather than depth is emphasized (LoBiondo-Wood and Haber, 1998).

Qualitative research

The naturalistic approach differs in underlying philosophical beliefs, in that it is based on the belief that there is no single objective reality, but that we all develop our own subjective reality; hence there is an increased focus on feelings, experiences, thoughts and interactions. Originating from social scientists, the naturalist research approach, often referred to as qualitative research, is concerned with the development of theory (induction) rather than the testing of theory (deduction). The acceptance and value recognition of qualitative research in medicine have been somewhat slow, although in recent years there has been an increasing number of publications of qualitative research in highly regarded medical science literature, suggesting a shift in acknowledgment and appreciation of what qualitative research may convey.

The strength of quantitative research lies in its ability to produce large-scale data, which can be tested for reliability and validity, and consequently can be generalized to a number of settings. The strength of qualitative research lies in its validity or intimacy with the truth and its ability to explore depths of meanings (Greenhalgh, 2001). In contrast to quantitative research, rather than focusing on a single aspect of measurement whereby certain elements of depth may be lost, qualitative research illuminates the experience in an attempt to understand its depth. In nursing much of the published nursing research lies within this paradigm, perhaps because nursing itself is concerned moreover with a holistic approach to individualized patient-centred care, which some may argue is more congruent with nursing philosophy (Munhall, 1982). It is important to recognize, however, the limitations of a foundation of knowledge based in its entirety on small-scale, non-generalizable studies, and there have been calls for a move towards an eclectic approach.

Contrary to experimental research, which tends to produce large-scale and often depersonalized data (Parahoo, 1997, p. 209), the numbers of participants are generally kept small, with the concern being more with the depth and richness of information than the quantity of participants and hence statistical power. Informants/participants are usually selected on the basis that they have experienced the phenomenon and are thus more able to shed light on this, which differs from the random or representative sample needed within quantitative studies. Sampling methods include purposive/theoretical sampling, convenience/opportunistic sampling and snowballing (Table 11.2). As a result of the limited size of the sample, it is important to recognize the limitations in relation to generalizability to other settings and patients.

Table 11.2 Sampling methods for qualitative research

Purposive sampling/ Theoretical sampling	Researcher deliberately chooses the sample on the basis of known characteristics, e.g. patients may be selected on the basis that they have experienced a certain phenomenon and thus can provide insight to the investigation. Theoretical sampling continues according to the data generated, searching for new data to develop theory until no new data emerge
Convenience/ Opportunistic sampling	The researcher chooses the sample simply as the opportunity presents itself, e.g. easy to recruit, likely to want to participate
Snowball sampling	Arises from convenience sampling, but gathers further participants through introduction to others known to them who are also in the group of interest

Qualitative research is particularly useful where there is no prior knowledge, and a need to generate theory; hence research using a qualitative approach will generally begin with a broad topic of investigation and, as the research progresses, the researcher begins to narrow the focus of research as the phenomenon is uncovered.

Popay and Williams (1998, p. 34) describe qualitative research as 'focusing on the meanings that people attach to experience, the relationship between knowledge, experience and action and the social factors that shape these processes'. Within qualitative research the uniqueness of individuals is expressed and the researcher seeks to uncover and understand this uniqueness through immersion in the social context. Critics might argue that through this immersion qualitative researchers fail to recognize the impact that they themselves have on the participants and, consequently, the researcher must constantly be aware of the possible influences of researcher bias and remain neutral. It is important to recognize that qualitative research is often criticized for its subjectivity and lack of scientific rigour; hence, it is particularly important to pay attention to research design, and method of data collection and analysis, and to provide sufficient detail to enable external assessment by others. Indeed, Koch (1996, p. 177) suggests that the resolution of issues of rigour should be the 'current pre-occupation' for qualitative researchers.

Data collection methods are generally guided by the question and the philosophical framework and principles adopted by the researcher. Most commonly data collection occurs through either in-depth/unstructured interviews, semi-structured interviews, observation and field notes, focus groups, diaries or examination of documentation. To capture the entirety of the data during interview techniques, the researcher generally tape-records the participant sessions. The enormity of data recorded should not be underestimated because the volumes of data will take considerable time to transcribe and analyse. A 1-hour interview can take up to 2–4 hours to transcribe.

Analysis of the data usually follows using a step-by-step approach, which generally involves the identification of themes and categories. Various techniques for data analysis have been described (Colaizzi, 1978; Van Manen, 1990). Computer software is available to assist in the analysis of the contents of the transcripts, such as NUD.IST (Richards and Richards, 1990). As mentioned earlier, one of the main criticisms of qualitative research is the lack of attention to rigour during the data collection and analysis phases. Importantly the researcher should seek to enhance reliability of the data through involvement of independent assessors, which ensures that the researcher has not overinterpreted or misinterpreted data. Validation strategies sometimes involve checking back with the participants to confirm with them that the themes reflect their experiences and interpretations (Mays and Pope, 1995), although O'Mahony (2001) highlights the potential difficulties with this, particularly if the participants have revealed difficult painful memories; therefore this should be carefully planned.

Final presentation of the data should be considered in order to exhibit the themes or categories with accompanying text examples demonstrating how these were developed and how the associated meanings or interpretations were attained. Data should be presented authentically and should enable the reader to follow the decision pathways and interpretations of the researcher so that the reader may assess the trustworthiness of the data.

As in quantitative research there are a variety of different approaches/philosophical underpinnings to qualitative research. Three approaches are demonstrated to include grounded theory, phenomenology and ethnography although these by no means describe the full diversity of qualitative methods:

Grounded theory

This was developed and described by Glaser and Strauss (1967). Grounded theorists search to uncover the 'social processes present in human interaction' (Cutliffe, 2000). Where there is little known about the phenomena or processes, grounded theory enables the development of a theory and goes beyond the mere description of a situation. Theoretical development occurs through constant comparison of data and is characterized by a non-linear process in which the researcher constantly revisits the data for constant comparatives, differences, similarities and patterns; hence data collection and analysis usually occur simultaneously. Unlike the unstructured interview process in phenomenology, the researcher using grounded theory will often adopt a variety of data collection methods to ensure that the study is grounded in data (Wimpenny and Gass, 2000). Data collection continues until it is completely saturated with no new concepts/categories emerging, so there are therefore no limitations to the numbers of participants. Sampling processes also differ in grounded theory in that the sampling is motivated by the emerging theory, hence 'theoretical sampling' (Cutliffe, 2000) rather than the 'purposeful' sampling usually used in phenomenology, although most researchers presently use the terms 'theoretical' and 'purposeful' interchangeably, so this does lead to some confusion for the reader. Several authors have discussed and highlighted the difficulties with method slurring, which is not uncommon within the literature (Baker et al., 1992; Wimpenny and Gass, 2000).

Example of grounded theory (Thomas and Retsas, 1999)

Purpose of the study

To construct a grounded theory that explains how the spirituality of people with terminal cancer develops as they make sense of and come to terms with their diagnosis.

Sample

Nineteen patients were purposively sampled, selected on the basis that they could provide insight into the phenomena being studied, which was developed by 'snowballing', e.g. by one person introducing another to the study.

Data collection

In-depth interviews, with guided questions that were modified during the course of the data collection. Follow-up interviews were conducted to debrief the participants and clarify data and insights.

Analysis

Constant comparative method of analysis described by Strauss and Corbin (1990).

Findings

This study found that people with terminal cancer develop a spiritualness, as they make sense of and come to terms with their diagnosis. In seeking self-preservation, three interconnected behaviours were identified, i.e. 'taking it all in', 'getting on with it' and 'putting it all together'. 'Taking it all in' involved the response and questioning of the diagnosis. 'Getting on with things' was when the participants were more able to confront the reality of their diagnosis and when they began to confront their cancer and mobilize by connecting with self, others, God or a higher being. 'Putting it all together' reflected how participants created meaning in their terminal cancer, and began to discover their 'self', taking stock of their life, changing their outlook, transforming, becoming spiritual and expanding their consciousness.

Learning

Transacting self-preservation is made complete as the person reaches a deeper level of understanding of self that is imbued with spiritual growth. It gives deep meaning and richness to the person's life as he or she transcends everyday experiences in the journey to death. The authors suggest that nurses must recognize that people with terminal cancer need help to find spiritual meaning. They suggest that 'nurses' spiritual support may mean nothing more than taking the time to provide physical and psychological caring that touches the spirit'. They highlight that some patients may find it difficult to articulate their spirituality.

Phenomenology

During the past two decades there has been increasing interest in the use of phenomenological research published within the nursing literature; however, varied interpretations of the original philosophical assumptions underpinning this approach have led to much criticism (Koch, 1995; Paley, 1997; Van der Zalm and Bergum, 2000). Phenomenology as described by Husserl (1859-1938) is the study of the 'lived experience' whereby the researcher aims to uncover or illuminate the real meaning of human lived experience by asking questions such as 'can you tell me what it is like to have been given a diagnosis of cancer?'. In Husserlian phenomenology, importantly, the researcher aims to 'bracket' any prior preconceptions in an attempt truly to reflect and describe the world as viewed by the participant. Koch (1996, p. 176) suggests that 'the hallmark of any genuinely phenomenological inquiry is that its task is a matter of describing'. Heidegger, a student of Husserl, later developed the original concepts of Husserl, placing greater importance on understanding the 'meanings' attached to the experience of individuals. He rejected the notion of 'bracketing', suggesting that one cannot separate the description from one's own interpretation and hence, during the data analysis, the prior experiences of the researcher are merged with the participant's data (Koch, 1996).

Ultimately the primary objective of phenomenological research is to describe and provide an understanding of a person's lived experience: 'instead of pin-pointing a minute segment of experience as in quantitative research, the phenomenological view enlarges the experience and attempts to understand it in the complexity of its context' (Thibodeau and MacRae, 1997). This is done through the use of in-depth interviews with the overall purpose of the data analysis process being to maintain the originality and demonstrate rigour.

Example of a phenomenological study (Breaden, 1997)

Purpose

Using hermeneutic phenomenology, this study examined the experiences of women who had all finished treatment and who were at least 8 months post-cancer diagnosis.

Sample size

Six women.

Data collection

In-depth interviews each lasting approximately an hour.

Analysis

After analysis of transcripts from in-depth interviews, return visits were made to the participants to discuss individual transcripts. Using the process of thematic analysis described by Van Manen (1990), the transcripts were read and reread several times to get a sense of the whole. This occurred during on-going data collection to enable the researcher to ask more focused questions. A highlighting approach was used to isolate thematic statements. Statements relating to the experience of surviving cancer were isolated and recurring themes were identified.

Issues of rigour

The participants were revisited for clarification of meanings. Dependability and confirmability were attempted through the use of a reflective journal.

Findings

Original text was used to demonstrate the construction of themes. Women describe a survival process that includes 'feeling whole again', 'the body as a house of suspicion', 'the future in question', 'changes in time', 'lucky to be alive' and 'sharing the journey'.

Comments

Although the researcher suggests that data analysis occurred simultaneously with data collection to enable the researcher to ask more focused questions, arguably in keeping with phenomenological principles interviews are generally unstructured, e.g. Koch (1996, p. 1979) states: 'I do not ask specific questions; the exchange is entirely open'. Despite using a reflective journal, it is unclear from the publication how this information was used and how it informed the analysis process, which would have been helpful to ascertain the trustworthiness of the data.

Ethnography

The primary purpose of ethnographic studies is to understand human behaviour and its relationship to the culture and social context in which it occurs (Hammersley and Atkinson, 1983). Ethnography can be defined as the systematic process of observing, detailing, describing, documenting and analysing the behaviours of cultural groups. To do this, the researcher enters the world of the group of interest to see it through the eyes of the individuals within the culture, and uses various methods of data collection, which usually include participant field observation as well as face-to-face interviews and recording of interactive dialogue within the cultural setting. Analysis occurs simultaneously in 'field' and involves the analysis of language, behaviour and field notes to make sense of the respondents' behaviour (Parahoo, 1997).

Example of an ethnographic study (Cope, 1995)

Purpose

To investigate the function of a breast cancer support group as perceived by the participants.

Sample

A convenience sample of 15 women diagnosed with breast cancer, all of whom were attending a cancer support group.

Data collection

Participant observation, plus two key informant interviews to seek further clarification, explanation and validation of the data.

Analysis

Content analysis of audio-tape recordings from 10 meetings and from the two key informants. Credibility was addressed through validation of the data by the informants. Auditability/reliability was checked through an independent review of the analysis process by an experienced researcher.

Findings

Three major categories were formed which described the purpose and benefits that the patients thought belonged to the group. These included exchanging information, sharing the illness experience and providing strength. All three categories were described by the researcher, and evidence was provided for each category.

Learning

Nurses should be cognizant of the functions of a breast cancer support group so that this information can be shared with women.

Conclusion

Although this chapter has dedicated itself to an overview of research methodology, the effect of research on the patient should be given precedence. We must make sure that patients are well informed and safe, and that participation is voluntary (Entwistle et al., 2002). Any research that involves patients should have prior ethical committee approval. Madsen et al. (2002) and Cox (1999) highlight the complex psychological processes experienced by patients in decision-making about participation, particularly in relation to experimental treatments. One way of maximizing acceptability to patients is to involve them in the initial design, so that the patient perspective can be encompassed.

Many patients are asked to participate in some of the national trials and as nurses we should endeavour to offer support and information to patients in their decision-making processes. Jenkins and Fallowfield (2000) report that less than 5% of patients are currently recruited to clinical trials in the UK. Naturally, if we are to advance knowledge further about cancer treatments, this figure must be improved. Jenkins and Fallowfield (2000) suggest that non-participation can be influenced by both the physician and the patient. Equally it would not be surprising if nurses also play some part in influencing patients. Consequently, not only is there a need to have a basic understanding of research methodology, but also to keep up to date with the current clinical trials in our specialist areas.

In summary, research has a crucial part to play in the development of nursing care and treatment for patients with cancer. This chapter outlined a range of methodological designs and, although both quantitative and qualitative research have been presented independently of each other, there may be advantages in combining these methodological approaches. Sadly, in preparing this chapter there was much evidence of poorly designed nursing research with little attention to rigour within the literature. It is essential therefore that, if we are to gain recognition for our contribution to research and knowledge, we seek to redress this by ensuring that any research that we as nurses undertake is well designed to give meaningful results.

CHAPTER 12

Research ethics relating to cancer

DAVID CARPENTER

Research is surely a good thing; it is not immediately obvious that there are any ethical considerations beyond some sort of imperative to undertake it. After all, there would be no reliably effective treatment and care were it not for research and the evidence base of health-care interventions would simply not exist. Effective cancer care and treatment, perhaps more than any other discipline, rely on previous and current research and we hope that future endeavours will provide hitherto elusive, curative treatment for some of the most serious cancers. Although strongly supporting research, this chapter aims to elucidate necessary limits on the enterprise. These limits may be identified by considering issues such as the motives of the researcher, the value of the research and, most importantly, the welfare of participants. In simple terms, these limits highlight the differences between research (which might actually provide extremely useful knowledge) and *ethical* research.

Ethical research is, ideally, altruistically motivated and worthwhile, and ensures the welfare of participants. These ideals are seldom fully attainable and the purpose of ethical review of research proposals is to assess the degree to which they are compromised and whether the proposed study falls within acceptable limits. It is likely that many readers will be considering undertaking a research project, probably as part of undergraduate or postgraduate study. The primary purpose of such a study will be the award of a degree: hardly an altruistic motive. It is also highly likely that the project will be small scale with little potential to provide any significant benefit to participants or others in the future. Although it might be unlikely that any participants will suffer significant harm, they will necessarily have to give their time and energy. To put the matter bluntly, students often *use* patients to gain a degree.

It is this issue of using people, albeit in the pursuit of valuable knowledge, that makes research ethically sensitive. Health-care research poses some of the greatest concerns, given that in most cases participants are sick, and in some cases they might be critically ill or dying. Cancer patients are often in these latter categories. Is it defensible to use them to gain knowledge, particularly when they, as participants, might gain little or no benefit and, indeed, might suffer considerable harm? Of course, the answer to this question is 'it all depends'. It depends on the skill of the researcher, the value of the research and the risks posed to the participants. Again, it is the purpose of ethical review to establish whether the proposed research satisfies the 'it all depends' criteria alluded to above.

This chapter goes on to consider research ethics from the perspectives of, first, the researcher, second, the research and, third, the participant. It will include an overview of the nature and roles of research ethics committees, particularly NHS Research Ethics Committees (NHSRECs). Before embarking on this enterprise, however, it is worth reflecting on some historical and some surprisingly recent examples of unethical research.

Unethical research

Kennedy and Grubb (2000) suggest that the greatest incentive to regulate health-care research was awareness of the atrocities committed during World War II in the name of medical research. According to Evans and Evans (1996) 23 doctors were convicted at the Nuremberg trials. Their deeds included: freezing subjects in an attempt to discover the most effective means of treating hypothermia; deliberately infecting subjects with malaria with an aim of discovering suitable vaccines; and inflicting and subsequently infecting wounds to test the efficacy of sulfanilamide as an antibacterial agent. Not surprisingly, many of the subjects died; all suffered immeasurably. The research did, however, provide useful knowledge and the doctors were able to provide more effective treatment for German troops. It is a chilling fact that valuable knowledge can be obtained relatively easily if researchers have no concern for the welfare of their subjects.

The doctors concerned were found guilty of crimes against humanity, and of fundamental breaches of human rights. The Nuremberg Code followed as an attempt to regulate future research on humans. The Nuremberg Code has subsequently been replaced by the World Medical Association's Declaration of Helsinki (2000), which remains as a key regulator of medical research. International codes, declarations and treaties are typically used to protect human rights, but they necessarily require states to sign up to them in order to be effective. There is little to prevent the unethical researcher undertaking their investigations in non-subscribing countries, although they would certainly find difficulty publishing any results, valuable or otherwise. European citizens enjoy protection of fundamental human rights by virtue of the European Convention of Human Rights. The articles of the convention form part of the Human Rights Act 1998, which came into force in 2000. The rights of research participants are therefore protected by the duties of researchers as stated in the Declaration of Helsinki and by law.

Further protection to research participants in clinical trials, particularly children and mentally incapacitated people, is provided within a recent European Union Directive (2001). All member states are required to pass legislation incorporating the provisions of the directive into national law, to come into force in 2004. At the time of writing, this legislation is in the form of a draft Statutory Instrument currently laid before parliament. This will be the first piece of English legislation, albeit secondary, regulating some aspects of health-care research.

Despite theoretical protection of research participants there have been more recent examples of unethical research. According to an urgent communication from the Chief Medical Officer of Health (DoH, 2000f), volunteers who took part in trials at the Chemical and Biological Defence Establishment at Porton Down were to be offered a Medical Assessment Programme (MAP). This followed investigations by Wiltshire Constabulary after it received complaints by volunteers. It would appear that the volunteers were suffering unusual ill-health, which they were attributing to their participation in the trials.

Between the 1940s and 1980s some 20 000 servicemen volunteered to be exposed to low levels of mustard gas and nerve agents, including sarin. The communication reports the Ministry of Defence (MoD) as not having seen any evidence connecting ill-health with participation in the trials. In July 2001 (Anon, 2001) the government launched an independent medical investigation. By this time there was compelling evidence that some volunteers had received dangerous doses and, moreover, some claimed to have been duped into believing that they would be researching the common cold.

A public outcry followed exposure of practices in Bristol and Alder Hey children's hospitals (DoH, 1999). Organs and tissues were routinely retained, after post mortem examinations, for several purposes, including medical research; it later became clear that no significant research was undertaken. Although in some cases parents had signed consent forms, it transpired that they were not made explicitly aware of the implications of doing so. After this exposure, the Chief Medical Officer of Health (CMO) conducted a census

(DoH, 2000e) to establish the nature and volume of retained organs and tissues in NHS trusts and medical schools. Among his conclusions was recognition of the potential research value of organs and tissues from the dead, but he urged that this should not override the feelings of families and the need for informed consent.

A further outcry followed the discovery that 20 000 brains had been taken for research after post mortem examinations. An investigation was conducted by Her Majesty's Inspector of Anatomy, Dr Jeremy Metters, after Mrs Elaine Isaacs discovered that her late husband's brain had been removed *post mortem* and given to Manchester University, for research, without her consent. The Isaacs Report (DoH, 2003b) revealed the extent of the practice.

It is clear, then, that unethical research is not a matter to be consigned to distant history. Arguably the need for rigorous ethical review and monitoring has never been stronger.

The researcher

Most health-care researchers are health-care professionals or at least working under their direction. This situation gives rise to an interesting analysis with regard to duty. It would seem obvious that health-care professionals, including nurses, have a primary duty towards the patient as an individual; any research activity is likely to subordinate this duty to the wider interests of a greater population. In simple terms, the role of the nurse changes from duty-bound practitioner to researcher.

In the introduction to the Code of Professional Conduct, the Nursing and Midwifery Council (NMC, 2002) states:

As a registered nurse, midwife or health visitor you are personally accountable for your practice. In caring for patients and clients, you must:
- Respect the patient or client as an individual
- Obtain consent before you give any treatment or care
- Protect confidential information
- Co-operate with others in the team
- Maintain your knowledge and competence
- Be trustworthy
- Act to identify and minimise any risks to patients and clients

The NMC (2002) goes on to state:

These are the shared values of all the United Kingdom health care regulatory bodies.

It is important that the professional imperatives stated above are described as 'values'; had they been absolute duties, most would be breached in the course of research. Most research entails using data gained from individuals or groups of patients to interrogate hypotheses or construct theories. The results of research can then be used to benefit the wider population. A health-care researcher would simply not be respecting patients and clients *as individuals*.

Analysis of the list of values, stated above, raises further problems. If these values were viewed as absolute duties, there would be inevitable conflicts, e.g. it would be very difficult, if not impossible, to maintain knowledge and competence while continuing to respect patients as individuals. Equally it would be difficult to maintain knowledge and competence without accessing and analysing data that might otherwise be treated as confidential. The usual purpose of collecting confidential health-care data is to optimize individual care and treatment; using it in the context of research is clearly a departure from this primary purpose. How can these problems be solved? The short answer is that a complete solution is unlikely; however, acceptable compromises can result in ethical research. The nature of these compromises can be understood by investigating:

- The roles and duties of health-care practitioners
- The regulation of research activities
- The rights of participants.

The last two issues are addressed later; the first is dealt with in more detail at this stage.

Health-care regulatory bodies typically provide further guidance to practitioners with regard to research. The NMC (2000) has produced criteria for safe and ethical conduct of research, and states:

> You must always refer to the *Code of Professional Conduct*. This document provides the framework for all actions of registrants.
>
> As well as using these documents, you need to be sure that the research or clinical trial you are carrying out meets specific criteria. These are that:
> - the project must be approved by the LREC;
> - management approval must be gained where necessary;
> - arrangements for obtaining consent must be clearly understood by all those involved;
> - confidentiality must be maintained;
> - patients must not be exposed to unacceptable risks;
> - patients should be included in the development of proposed projects where appropriate;
> - accurate records must be kept and research questions need to be well structured and aimed at producing clearly anticipated care or service outcomes and benefits;

Given the overriding obligation to refer to the Code of Professional Conduct, it might be observed that the most compelling criteria are those requiring LREC and management approval for research; these are considered later.

Duties of health-care practitioners are wider than those prescribed by health-care regulatory bodies. Moral and legal duties ('moral' and 'ethical' can be treated as synonymous in normal discourse) are equally, if not more, significant. It is not *necessarily* the case that professional duties, as stated by professional regulatory bodies, are either legal or moral, although in most cases they will be. It might be argued that duties can be hierarchically ordered; if so, moral duties would be at the top of the hierarchy. Although exceptions are clearly possible, one would hope that the law is moral and that professional duties require practitioners to act both morally and legally.

What are the key moral duties relating to health-care research? It has already been argued that there is a moral duty to undertake research. It is uncontentious to claim that patients have an entitlement to the best possible care and treatment which necessarily entails research. If this is, however, the sole duty, it would be legitimate to pursue any activity having this as its goal. In short, patients and healthy volunteers could be used or abused with impunity, as illustrated in the earlier examples. Proposed research can be analysed with reference to theories of ethics. In simple terms, theories can be divided into those that relate to the motives of the moral agent and those that relate to acts.

Kantian ethics is possibly the best example of an agent-based or deontological theory (O'Neill, 1995). The agent is required to adhere to strict duties, e.g. not to lie. Kant starts from the question 'What ought I to do?' and searches for a supreme moral duty, which he calls the 'Categorical Imperative'. The categorical imperative, sometimes known as the 'golden rule', has been formulated in a variety of ways, the most common of which is: 'Act only on that maxim which at the same time you can will to be a universal law.' This maxim comes down to an obligation to 'do as you would be done by' and places the person at the heart of the theory. Kant reasons that, given that people are inclined to act morally and are therefore capable of moral activity, they are deserving of moral respect. For this reason, people should never be used as a means to an end; rather, they should be regarded as 'ends in themselves'.

The most superficial analysis of research activity reveals a need to use people as means to ends; this offends the fundamental basis of Kantian ethics. What of the research participant who freely volunteers to participate, as is often the case for patients with cancer when undergoing trials for new treatments? The Kantian position requires people to treat themselves with the same respect as they treat others; it is not acceptable to use oneself as a means to an end. Without further, increasingly complex argument, it can be concluded that no strong Kantian can readily approve of health-care research. It might also be concluded that any person of Kantian persuasion has a morally defensible ground for refusing to undertake or participate in human research.

Other moral theories relate to acts rather than the motives of the actor; the best known is utilitarianism (Goodin, 1995). Utilitarianism is an example of consequentialist ethics where the focus is on the consequences of actions, in other words ends. In determining the morality of an act the agent is required to evaluate its outcome with regard to the degree to which it promotes human interests, with a proviso that every individual's interest should be treated equally. Various forms of utilitarianism identify different individual interests; these include pleasure, happiness and, more recently, preferences and welfare. One of the main reasons for promoting human interests is human capacity to experience, e.g. pleasure and pain; in so far as other animals have this capacity, modern utilitarianism takes them into account. It is not always possible to promote positive outcomes, e.g. the greatest pleasure. In this case an action may be ethical in so far as it promotes positive and/or minimizes negative outcomes.

The moral defence of most health-care research lies in utilitarian reasoning. It may be acceptable to use a person, perhaps in a drugs trial, if the outcome is knowledge, which might be employed in achieving a greater good. But what if a greater good could be attained by abusing people, as in some of the examples of unethical research discussed earlier? This concern is sometimes advanced as a criticism of utilitarianism along with further concerns about accuracy of prediction of outcomes and relative merits of different interests. It is possible to employ utilitarianism when evaluating rules as well as acts. Although an act that promotes the welfare of a majority over the suffering of a minority might be considered moral, it is unlikely that many would agree that such a rule would be acceptable. Imagine a rule claiming that we *ought* to promote the welfare of the majority regardless of suffering caused to a minority. Such a rule is hardly calculated to promote overall human interests because we might all, with good reason, fear becoming part of that minority.

The ethical researcher, then, should be aiming to promote human interests and a proposed project will be ethical in so far as it is designed to do so. When considering the means to this end, most researchers will be confronted with a need to compromise some basic duties. The first priority is to establish whether it is absolutely necessary to compromise these duties. Second, it is important to minimize any potential harm or disadvantages that might arise. Third, where harm, albeit minimal, is inevitable, the researcher is obliged to muster a robust moral defence.

In the first case, a great deal might be achieved by accessing a research population to whom no primary professional duty is owed. Health-care practitioners frequently research their 'own' patients and clients, producing an inevitable conflict of duty. When challenged, it becomes clear that often the reason for this is simply convenience. Examples of the second case include provision of access to support organizations when respondents are interviewed on sensitive topics, e.g. 'living with cancer'. The administration of a placebo is a moral harm in so far as it is a deceit; it may also be a practical harm in that its consequence is deprivation of active treatment. The third obligation would be met in cases where there is no known alternative to the trial drug and it is at least possible that it will have no positive effects beyond that of a placebo or, more contentiously, that potential harms in the form of side effects might outweigh any benefit.

What are the legal duties of the researcher? Legal duties can be derived from statute law (acts of parliament) and case law. The most significant statute is the Human Rights Act 1998; all other law relating to health-care research should be read and interpreted in conjunction with it. In relation to health-care research, the most important provisions of the Act include rights to life, liberty and privacy, and prohibition of discrimination. Some of the examples of unethical research discussed earlier violate the right to life. Research participants' rights to liberty and privacy must be protected by ensuring that they are aware of any infringements resulting from research, and full consent is given. Law relating to consent is largely derived from case law and is considered later from the perspective of the participant.

The issue of discrimination is interesting. A clear example of discrimination arises when researchers select participants using inclusion criteria other than those that are scientifically defensible or designed to protect vulnerable people, e.g. prisoners might be selected on the grounds that they are easy to monitor. It is equally possible to discriminate by exclusion. Participating in therapeutic research allows the possibility of conferring benefit; if a person were excluded on the grounds of, for example, not speaking English, this would be discriminatory. Therapeutic research entails testing a form of treatment on a person who might benefit. It should be emphasized that benefit is only a possibility and, for this reason, the distinction between therapeutic and non-therapeutic research is arguable; the primary intention of the researcher, in both cases, is acquisition of knowledge rather than provision of treatment.

Another significant example of statute is the Data Protection Act 1998, which applies to all personal data identifying the participant. Researchers have duties to gain consent from the participant before accessing personal data, making it clear what the data will be used for. They are also obliged to anonymize any published data, thus ensuring the participant's right to privacy. If researchers wish to access patient data held by a trust, they must seek authorization from the data custodian, known as the Caldicott Guardian.

Having considered the duties of researchers in some detail, it is worthwhile enquiring whether they have any rights. The short answer is that they have the rights that are necessary to meet their duties, e.g. a right to apply to an NHS research ethics committee (REC). Researchers do not have a right to undertake research; arguably they have duties to extend existing knowledge. Legislation currently before parliament will afford researchers a legal right to a prompt response from an REC; this would normally be within 60 days (DoH, 2003c).

The research

The objective of health-care research is acquisition of knowledge, which enables provision of effective, evidence-based care and treatment. Conferring benefit on participants is rarely the immediate objective of the researcher as discussed earlier; the likelihood is that the outcomes of the research will be used for the benefit of others. Perhaps the exception to this general principle is action research where findings are continuously fed back into the field. In a typical randomized controlled clinical trial, participants enter a 'lottery' where they may or may not be allocated the trial drug, which may or may not be effective. Any benefit is largely a matter of chance. If, however, research proves a drug to be effective, there is normally an obligation to continue to provide it to all participants after the trial has concluded (World Medical Association, Declaration of Helsinki, 2000).

It is not difficult to understand why all health-care research must be ethically reviewed. Given the comparatively recent examples of unethical research, it is not surprising that the DoH has produced governance arrangements for research in the NHS. These arrangements are known as 'Governance Arrangements for Research Ethics Committees' (GAfREC) (DoH, 2001b). The DoH requires all NHS research to be reviewed by an NHS REC. NHS research is defined in

GAfREC as any research involving patients, relatives and carers, staff, access to data, organs and bodily material, and the use of NHS premises and facilities. It includes those who have recently died on NHS premises.

The primary purpose of RECs is to 'protect the dignity, safety and well-being of all actual or potential research participants' (DoH, 2001b). RECs do have a secondary role with regard to researchers, having consideration for their interests and, more importantly, their safety. Strictly speaking, RECs do not approve proposals because researchers ultimately require the approval of appropriate managers and professionals in the specific locations in which the research takes place. RECs may or may not provide a favourable opinion, a necessary requirement before commencement of any study.

RECs are established by health authorities and the DoH, but they are strictly independent and not in any way accountable to NHS trusts. This ensures that proposals can be reviewed freely in the absence of any sort of coercion. The membership of RECs includes relevant health-care professionals, experts, e.g. a scientific officer with knowledge of statistical analysis, and laity. Lay members are particularly important given the likelihood that they will be more able to review a proposal from the participant's perspective. At least a third of the membership must comprise laity. There is an obligation for all members to undertake introductory and continuing training. It should be noted that membership of an REC is entirely voluntary.

Where a study is to be conducted over five or more sites, an application is normally made to a multicentre REC (MREC) for review; in other cases it is reviewed by a local REC (LREC). The effect of EU Directive 2001/20/E, however, is such that the favourable opinion of one REC is sufficient to allow research to take place in other localities. The task of other LRECs is limited to evaluating the proposal with regard to locality issues, including consideration of resources and availability of a local, suitably qualified researcher.

An application to an REC should be viewed as one of the last stages before commencement of a project. RECs expect complete documentation providing evidence that the project has been peer reviewed or, in the case of a small-scale student project, that it is appropriately supervised. Where necessary, applications should also provide evidence that the proposal has received the support of the relevant trust's research and development department, i.e. it has management approval. It is equally important to provide evidence of compliance with the provisions of the Data Protection Act 1998.

In summary, in order to gain the favourable opinion of an REC, proposed research must meet the conditions stated above and:

- comply with the Declaration of Helsinki
- comply with European and national law
- demonstrate that the researcher has met her moral, legal and professional duties
- meet the criteria stated in sections 9.13–9.18 of GAfREC (DoH, 2001b).

The participant

It should now be clear that participating in research is likely to be, at least in part, an act of altruism. Direct benefit to research participants is unlikely to be a primary endpoint of many research projects, although there are, of course, exceptions. Mostly, any benefits accrued will be a matter of chance and most participants will find themselves suffering some disadvantage in the interests of health-care advancement. The welfare of all participants is obviously important, but it should be noted that there is a real danger that some people who are suffering from the most serious conditions, including some cancers, may see themselves as having little to lose. These people, along with other vulnerable individuals, including minors and people experiencing mental disorders, are particularly in need of protection.

When considering the welfare of participants, an obvious starting point is to enquire whether or not the research is necessary and worthwhile. The DoH (2001c) states:

> It is essential that existing sources of evidence, especially systematic reviews, are considered carefully prior to undertaking research. Research which duplicates other work unnecessarily or which is not of sufficient quality to contribute something useful to existing knowledge is in itself unethical.

This stance undoubtedly jeopardizes many student projects that aim to employ primary data collection; however, it is difficult to argue that the interests of participants can reasonably be subordinated to the interests of students. Research based on secondary data or simply designing a potential project will meet most reasonable learning outcomes.

Worthwhile research should, wherever possible, be designed to minimize risks and disadvantages to participants. A good example of such a strategy is the decision to use a control arm only when it is absolutely necessary. Participants acting as controls usually receive placebo 'treatment' or no treatment at all. Although they avoid risks associated with the trial treatment, they may suffer as a result of being deprived of an alternative, active treatment.

Research that has been well designed may still pose risks to participants. In this case it is essential to ensure that all participants are made fully aware of the implications of their participation. They should be given clear information with sufficient time to reflect on it and opportunities to discuss it with others. Consent is an absolute requirement and that consent should be real. To meet English legal obligations, it must be freely given, in the absence of any sort of inducement and in the light of sufficient information, and the participant must have the mental capacity to understand the implications of their participation. All participants must be assured that their (continuing) participation is entirely voluntary and without prejudice to any normal care and treatment that they might otherwise receive.

Similarly, well-designed research may still entail the collection of sensitive data and other material, including tissue, which might have serious implications for the participant. The nature of data collected must be made explicit to the participant whose privacy must be safeguarded as far as possible; this may be achieved by collecting the minimum data necessary and, subsequently, treating it in confidence. Participant confidentiality is protected by the legal and professional duties discussed earlier.

Ethical considerations of participants can be identified in relation to key stages of the research process, including:

* identification of potential participants
* recruitment of participants
* informing participants
* gaining participants' consent.

Research participants are typically identified using inclusion and exclusion criteria determined by the scientific design of the study. There are, however, overriding ethical concerns. Unless they are necessarily participants of the particular study, it is normal to exclude vulnerable people. Vulnerable people include those who are seriously ill, those whose freedoms are compromised and people lacking capacity. It is normal, then, to exclude terminally ill people, prisoners, minors, people with serious mental disorders, and any other person who does not have the capacity to understand the nature and implications of their involvement, i.e. any person who cannot realistically consent to participation. Some research does involve vulnerable people; how could effective care and treatment for this group be provided without some research directly involving them?

In the case of therapeutic research where there is at least a chance of potential benefit, it is possible, with REC approval, to undertake research in the absence of explicit consent. A person holding parental responsibility for a minor can consent on his or her behalf although, given the provisions of the Children Act 1989, they should assure themselves that the welfare interests of the minor are not jeopardized. There is no provision in English law for proxy consent in the case of adults, although a relative could provide assent if appropriate. The issue of non-therapeutic research is more contentious. An REC can approve research involving vulnerable people in non-therapeutic research, as long as any risks incurred are minimal and all reasonable steps have been taken to protect the interests of the participants, including respecting confidentiality.

Participants should be invited to join a study, i.e. they should be given the opportunity to opt in. It is unethical to require participants to opt out. This basic requirement is easily breached. An example might be sending a postal questionnaire to a potential participant and requiring them to inform the researcher if they do not wish to participate. Furthermore, imagine the potential distress arising from receiving a questionnaire including sensitive topics, without any prior warning. In most cases it is normal to send a letter of invitation with an accompanying information sheet seeking the participant's agreement to join a study. Potential participants may, of course, be approached directly or through a third party; in any event, comprehensible information, ideally in writing, is an absolute requirement. When a questionnaire is directly administered, information may be given orally or may comprise an introductory paragraph on the questionnaire itself. The Central Office for Research Ethics Committees (COREC) provides templates for information sheets and consent forms. These can be easily accessed via the office's website at www.corec.org.uk. It should be noted that information sheets and consent forms must be on headed paper, include dates and version numbers, and provide the researcher's contact details.

The reason why information is so important is that real consent is dependent on it. Consent, again, is an absolute requirement. Consent need not necessarily be in writing, e.g. completion and return of a simple questionnaire by an informed participant may reasonably be taken as evidence of consent. In most cases, written consent will be necessary. It is normally taken at the time of participation by the researcher, who must ensure that the participant has had sufficient time to consider the implications of involvement. A consent form must include evidence of the participant's general willingness to join the study based on information received, their rights to withdraw without negative consequences, and explicit consent where sensitive data are collected. Examples of the last include photographs, video and audio recordings, data from medical records, and data derived from tissue and other specimens. Participants must be informed of the overall management of the data, e.g. audio recordings are normally transcribed but the original tape is either destroyed or erased. Any data or other material retained for future use must be brought to the attention of the participant. The most contentious example in this category is retained tissue.

Retained tissue is particularly significant in research on cancer care and treatment. Tumour cells are frequently collected in the course of therapeutic and non-therapeutic research; in the former, research can be conducted to find the most effective chemotherapeutic regimen, thus directly benefiting the patient. In the latter, retained cells can be used in the course of developing drugs that might benefit others, possibly at a time long after the death of the patient. This use might well be commercial. Given concerns raised by the unethical retention of organs and tissue, discussed earlier, the DoH (2003a) has issued an interim statement on the use of human organs and tissue. The statement provides guidance while necessary changes are made to existing law. Briefly, no tissue may be retained without the explicit, voluntary consent of the patient; the purpose of retention must be made clear and the tissue should be treated as a donation. In effect patients forfeit any property rights to the tissue. Tissue may be used commercially but it must be retained within the EU. Although tissue is normally anonymized, there are typically coded links such that, in the event of significant information coming to light, it is possible to contact the donor.

The importance of research involving tissue donated by cancer patients cannot be overstated. It is worth noting that the unethical retention of organs and tissue in the past could negatively impact on this research because potential donors or their relatives may have serious concerns. This is perhaps one of the most compelling grounds for ensuring that research is always ethical.

One final ethical issue remains. At the beginning of this chapter, it was argued that research is ethically sensitive because it frequently entails the use of people for the benefit of others. No benefit can be gained unless the results of research are successfully disseminated. On this ground, publication of research is a moral duty. In other words, the endpoint of valuable research should never be simply the award of a degree or promotion of personal or institutional status.

Glossary

Allele One of several alternative forms of a gene occupying the same locus on a chromosome.

Angiogenesis Formation of new blood vessels.

Apoptosis Programmed cell death.

ATP Adenosine triphosphate.

Cancer Uncontrolled proliferation and growth of cells into other tissues.

CDK Cyclin-dependent kinases.

Cell Basic unit of all living matter.

Cellular senescence Limited capacity of cells to divide beyond a finite number of population doublings.

CFCs Chlorofluorocarbons.

Chromatin DNA-protein complex containing genes in the cell.

Codon Three adjacent nucleotides in a nucleic acid that code for one amino acid.

Deoxyribose The five carbon sugar with hydrogen at the 2' position found in DNA. Different from the ribose sugar found in RNA.

Diploid A cell containing two sets of chromosomes – the number found in normal somatic cells.

DNA Deoxyribonucleic acid.

DNA ligase An enzyme that seals together two DNA fragments.

DNA polymerase An enzyme that links complementary nucleotides together to replicate DNA.

Endoplasmic reticulum Series of inter-connecting tubular tunnels in the cell.

Epigenetic Non-genetic changes that alter an organism's phenotype, such as methylation.

Eukaryotic An animal or plant that has a membrane-bound nucleus and organelles.

Exons A segment of DNA that is expressed by a mature RNA product.

Germ cell Precursor cells that give rise to sperm or eggs.

Germline The lineage of germ cells, as distinct from somatic cells.

Golgi apparatus A structure that modifies proteins and fats in the cell.

HAMAs Human anti-mouse monoclonal antibodies.

Haploid Cells containing only one set of chromosomes – usually germ cells (e.g. sperm and eggs)

IHC Immunohistochemistry.

Introns Non-coding DNA sequences separating the coding exons. During gene expressions introns are removed from mature RNA by splicing.

Locus Site of a gene on a chromosome.

LREC Local research ethics committee.

Lysosomes Spherical bodies containing digestive enzymes in the cell.

mAB Monoclonal antibody.

Metastasis Spread of a primary cancer to another part of the body.

Mitochondria Bodies that break down sugar molecules in the presence of oxygen and produce energy in the form of ATP in the cell.

Mitosis Cell division.

MMPs Matrix metalloproteins.

Monogenic Controlled by, or associated with a single gene.

MREC Multicentre research ethics committee.

Nuclear envelope Double-layered membrane protecting and separating the nucleus from the cytoplasm and molecules in the cell.

Nucleolus Part of cell nucleus and produces ribosomes.

Nucleosome A structural unit of chromatin.

Nucleotide The basic subunits of nucleic acids. Constructed from pyrimidine or purine base, a pentose sugar and a phosphate group.

Organelle Subcellular functional components of a cell, e.g. the nucleus.

PCR Polymerase chain reaction.

Pentose A sugar containing five carbon molecules.

Polygenic Controlled by, or associated with, more than one gene.

Promoter A site on DNA that is upstream (5') to the coding sequence, to which the RNA polymerase enzymes bind, and transcription of which will be initiated.

PSA Prostate-specific antigen.

Ribose A pentose sugar found in the nucleotides of RNA.

Ribosomes Organelles made of rRNA and protein. These are the protein-making machinery.

RNA Ribonucleic acid.

Somatic cell All cells of an organism except those of the germline.

Splicing Removal of introns from unprocessed RNA molecule.

Transcription Process whereby RNA is created from DNA template.

Translation Synthesis of protein from genetic information held in an mRNA molecule.

Translational oncology Applying cancer research to clinical practice.

References

Abgrall S, Orbach D, Bonhomme-Faivre L, Orbach-Arbous S (2002) Tumours in organ transplant recipients may give clues to their control by immunity. Anticancer Research 22(6b): 3597-3604.

Adams J, Carder PJ, Downey S et al. (2000)Vascular endothelial growth factor (VEGF) in breast cancer: comparison of plasma, serum, and tissue vegf and microvessel density and effects of tamoxifen 1. Cancer Research 60: 2898-2905.

Alberts B, Bray D, Lewis J, Raff M, Roberts K, Watson JD (1994) Internal organisation of the cell. In: Molecular Biology of the Cell, 3rd edn. New York: Garland Publishing.

Allen RE (1990) The Concise Oxford Dictionary of Current English, 8th edn. Oxford: Clarendon Press.

Altfeld M, Rosenberg ES (2000) The role of CD4+ T helper cells in the cytotoxic T lymphocyte response to HIV. 12: 375-380.

American Society of Clinical Oncology (ASCO) (1996) Clinical practice guidelines for the use of tumor markers in breast and colorectal cancer. Journal Clinical Oncology 14: 2843-2877.

ASCO (1998) 1997 update and recommendations for the use of tumor markers in breast and colorectal cancer. Journal Clinical Oncology 16: 793-795.

American Urological Association (2000) Prostate-specific antigen (PSA) best practice policy. Oncology 14: 267-272, 277-2778, 280 et seq. (www.cancernetwork.com/journals/oncology; accessed Nov 2002).

Andre FT (2003) Vaccinology: past achievements, present roadblocks and future promises. Vaccine 21: 593-595.

Andreeff M, Goodrich DW, Pardee AB (2000) Cell proliferation, differentiation, and apoptosis. In: Bast RC Jr, Kufe DW, Pollock RE, et al. (eds), Cancer Medicine, 5th edn. Hamilton, Ont: BC Decker.

Anon (2001) Porton Down probe launched. The Guardian 30 July 2001

Antequera F, Boyes J, Bird A (1990) High levels of de novo methylation and altered chromatin structure at CpG islands in cell lines. Cell 62: 503-514.

Appay V, Rowland-Jones SL (2002) Premature aging of the immune system: the cause of AIDS? Trends in Immunology 23: 580-585.

Armstrong AC, Hawkins RE (2001) Vaccines in oncology: background and clinical potential. British Journal of Radiology 74: 991-1002.

Armstrong K, Eisen A, Weber B (2000) Assessing the risk of breast cancer. New England Journal of Medicine 342: 564-571.

Association of Clinical Biochemists in Ireland (1999) Guidelines for the Use of Tumor Markers (www.iol.ie/_deskenny/ acbi.html; accessed Oct 2002).

Avery OT, Macleod CM, McCarty M (1944) Studies on the chemical nature of the substance introducing transformation of pneumococcal types. Journal of Experimental Medicine 79: 137–158.

Baildam A, Keeling F, Noble M, Thompson L, Bundred N, Hopwood P (2001) Nurse led follow-up for women treated for breast cancer: a randomised controlled trial. European Journal of Surgical Oncology 27: 792.

Baker C, Wuest J, Norager-Stern P (1992) Method slurring: the grounded theory/phenomenology example. Journal of Advanced Nursing 17: 1355–1360.

Balmain A (2001) Cancer genetics: from Boveri and Mendel to microarrays. National Review of Cancer 1(1): 77–82.

Baselga J, Albanell J (2001) Mechanism of action of anti-HER-2 monoclonal antibodies. Annals of Oncology 12(suppl 1): S35–S41.

Baselga J, Norton L, Albanell J, Kim YM, Mendelsohn J (1998). Recombinant humanized anti-HER-2 antibody (Herceptin) enhances the anti-tumour activity of paclitaxel and doxorubicin against HER-2/neu overexpressing human breast cancer xenografts. Cancer Research 58: 2825–2831.

Bast RC, Ravdin P, Hayes DF et al. (2001) 2000 update of recommendations for the use of tumor markers in breast and colorectal cancer: clinical practice guidelines of the American Society of Clinical Oncology [Erratum]. Journal of Clinical Oncology 19: 4185–4188; 20(8): 2213.

Baylin SB, Herman JG (2000) DNA hypermethylation in tumourigenesis. Trends in Genetics 16: 168–174.

Baylin SB, Belinsky SA, Herman JG (2000) Aberrant methylation of gene promoters in cancer – concepts, misconcepts, and promise. Journal of the National Cancer Institute 92: 1460–1461.

Becknell B, Caligiuri MA (2003) Cancer T cell therapy expands. Nature Medicine 9: 257–258.

Bell R (2002) Duration of therapy in metastatic breast cancer: management using Herceptin. Anticancer Drugs 12: 561–568.

Berd D (1998) Cancer vaccines: reborn or just recycled? Seminars in Oncology 25: 605–610.

Berd D (2001) Autologous, hapten-modified vaccine as treatment for human cancers. Vaccine 19: 2565–2570.

Berger MS, Leopold LH, Dowell JA, Korth-Bradley JM, Sherman ML (2002) Licensure of gemtuzumab ozogamicin for the treatment of selected patients 60 years of age and older with acute myeloid leukemia in first relapse. Investigational New Drugs 20: 395–406.

Bidart JM, Thuillier F, Augereau C et al. (1999) Kinetics of serum tumor marker concentrations and usefulness in clinical monitoring. Clinical Chemistry 45: 1690–1707.

Bird A (1992) The essentials of DNA methylation. Cell 70: 5–8.

Birmingham K (2002) What is translational oncology? Nature Medicine 8: 647.

Black N (1994) Why do we need qualitative research? Journal of Epidemiology and Community Health 48: 425–426.

Blagosklomy M (2002) From the war on cancer to translational oncology. Cancer Biology and Therapy July.

Bodey B, Bodey B Jr, Siegel S, Kiaser HE (2000) Failure of cancer vaccines: the significant limitations of this approach to immunotherapy. Anticancer Research 20: 2665-2676.

Bonfrer JMG, Duffy MJ, Radtke M et al. (1999) Tumor markers in gynaecological cancers: EGTM recommendations. Anticancer Research 19: 2807-2810.

Boon T, Van den Enbde B (2003) Tumour immunology. Current Opinion in Immunology 15: 129-130.

Bowling A (1997) Research Methods in Health: Investigating health and health services. Milton Keynes, Buckingham: Open University Press.

Bowling A (2001) Measuring Disease, 2nd edn. Milton Keynes, Buckingham: Open University Press.

Breaden K (1997) Cancer and beyond: the question of survivorship. Journal of Advanced Nursing 26: 978-984.

Breivik J, Gaudernack G (1999) Genomic instability, DNA methylation, and natural selection in colorectal carcinogenesis. Seminars in Cancer Biology 9: 245-254.

Bremers ATJ, Kuppen PJK, Parmiani G (2000) Tumour immunotherapy: the adjuvant treatment of the 21st century? European Journal of Surgical Oncology 26: 418-424.

Brennan P, Croft P (1994) Interpreting the results of observational research: chance is not such a fine thing. British Medical Journal 309,727-730.

British Medical Association (1997) Family Health Encyclopaedia. London: BMA Books.

Bromberg JE, Siemers MD, Taphoorn MJ (2002) Is a 'vanishing tumour' always a lymphoma? Neurology 59: 762-764.

Buckley RH (2003) 27.Transplantation immunology: organ and bone marrow. Journal of Allergy and Clinical Immunology 112(2 suppl): S733-744.

Burnet FM (1967) Immunological aspects of malignant disease. Lancet i: 1171-1174.

Burns EA, Leventhal (2000) Aging, immunity and cancer. Cancer Control 7: 513-522.

Cahill DP, Lengauer C, Yu J et al. (1998) Mutations of mitotic checkpoint genes in human cancers. Nature 392: 300-303.

Cancer Progress Report 2001 (2001) National Cancer Institute, NIH, DHMS, Bethesda, MD.

Cancer Research (2002a) Breast cancer. Retrieved from Cancer Research UK website (www.cancerresearchuk.org; accessed March 3 2003).

Cancer Research (2002b) Colorectal (bowel) cancer. Retrieved from Cancer Research UK website (www.cancerresearchuk.org; accessed March 3 2003).

Cancer Research (2002c) Lung cancer. Retrieved from Cancer Research UK website (www.cancerresearchuk.org; accessed March 3 2003).

CancerVOICES (2002) News, Views and action. CancerVOICES issue 7.

Cao Y, Lam L (2003) Bispecific antibody conjugate in therapeutics. Advanced Drug Delivery Reviews 55: 171-179.

Carter P, Presta L, Gorman CM et al. (1992) Humanization of an anti-p185HER-2 antibody for human cancer therapy. Proceedings of the National Academy of Sciences of the USA 89: 4285-4289.

Cartmel B, Reid M (2000) Cancer control and epidemiology. In: Greonwald S, Frogge M, Goodman M, Yarbro C (eds), Cancer Nursing: Principles and practice 5th edn. Boston, MA: Jones & Bartlett.

Cella D, Tulsky D, Gray G et al. (1993) The functional assessment of cancer therapy scale: development and validation of the general measure. Journal of Clinical Oncology 11: 570-579.

Chen J, Flurkey K, Harrison DE (2002) A reduced peripheral blood CD4+ lymphocyte proportion is a consistent ageing phenotype. Mechanisms Ageing and Development 13: 1445-153.

Cheson BD (2001) Some like it hot. Journal of Clinical Oncology 19: 3908-3911.

Cheung KL, Rosamund C, Graves L, Robertson JFR (2002) Autoantibodies as circulating cancer markers. In: Diamandis EP, Fritsche H, Schwartz MK, Chan DW (eds), Tumor Markers: Physiology, pathobiology, technology and clinical applications. Chicago: AACC Press, pp. 123-132.

Coghlan A (1991) The second chance for antibodies. New Scientist 19: 34-39.

Cohen M (1987) A historical overview of the phenomenological movement. Image: Journal of Nursing Scholarship 19: 31-34.

Colaizzi PF (1978) Psychological research as the phenomenologist views it. In: Valle R, King M (eds), Existential Phenomenological Alternatives for Psychology. Oxford: Oxford University Press, pp. 48-71.

Collins FS, Patrinos A, Jordan E, Chakravarti A, Gesteland R, Walters L (1998) New goals for the US Human Genome Project: 1998-2003. Science 282: 682-689.

Colvin DM (2000) Alkylating agents and platinum antitumor compounds. In: Bast Jr RC, Kufe DW, Pollock RE et al. Cancer Medicine, 5th edn. Hamilton, Ont: BC Decker.

Cook T, Reeves J, Lanigan A, Stanton P (2001) Her-2 as prognostic and predictive marker for breast cancer. Annals of Oncology 12(suppl 1): S23-S28.

Cope D (1995) Functions of a breast cancer support group as perceived by the participants: An ethnographic study. Cancer Nursing 18: 472-478.

Corner J (2001) What is cancer? In: Corner J, Bailey C (eds), Cancer Nursing: Care in context. Oxford: Blackwell Scientific.

Corner J (2002) Nurses' experiences of cancer. European Journal of Cancer Care 11: 193-199.

Cornwell J (1997) Cancer: the war against it. Sunday Times 1 June, pp14-19.

Costello RT, Fauriat C, Gastaut J-A, Olive D (2003) New approaches in the immunotherapy of haematological malignancies. European Journal of Haematology 70: 333-345.

Cox K (1998) Investigating psychosocial aspects of participation in early anti-cancer drug trials: towards a choice of methodology. Journal of Advanced Nursing 27: 488-496.

Cox K (1999) Researching research: patients' experiences of participation in phase 1 and II anti-cancer drug trials. European Journal of Oncology Nursing 3: 143-152.

Crawford J (2002) Pegfilgrastim administered once per cycle reduces incidence of chemotherapy-induced neutropenia (Review). Drug 62(suppl 1): 89-98.

Cutliffe J (2000). Methodological issues in grounded theory. Journal of Advanced Nursing 31: 1470-1484.

Davidson EJ, Kitchener HC, Stern PL (2002) The use of vaccines in the prevention and treatment of cervical cancer. Clinical Oncology 14: 193-200.

Davies CG, Gallo ML, Corvalan RF (1999). Transgenic mice as a source of fully human antibodies for the treatment of cancer. Cancer and Metastasis Review 18: 421-425.

Dearden C (2002) Monoclonal antibody therapy of haematological malignancies (Therapy review). Biodrugs 16: 283-301.

Department of Health (DoH) (1995) A Framework for Commissioning Cancer Services. London: DoH.

DoH (1999) The Royal Liverpool Children's Inquiry Report. London: The Stationery Office.

DoH (2000a) The NHS Cancer Plan. London: DoH.

DoH (2000b) Manual of Cancer Standards. London: DoH.

DoH (2000c) Towards a Strategy for Nursing Research and Development: Proposals for action. London: DoH.

DoH (2000d) The Nursing Contribution to Cancer Care. London: DoH.

DoH (2000e) Report of a Census of Organs and Tissues Retained by Pathology Services in England. London: The Stationery Office.

DoH (2000f) CEM/CMO/2000/15.

DoH (2001a) The NHS Cancer Plan: Making progress. London: DoH.

DoH (2001b) Governance Arrangements for Research Ethics Committees. London: The Stationery Office.

DoH (2002) National Patient Survey. London: DoH.

DoH (2003a) The Use of Human Organs and Tissue – An Interim Statement London: DoH.

DoH (2003b) The Isaacs Report. London: The Stationery Office.

DoH (2003c) The Medicines for Human Use (Clinical Trials) Regulations. London: DoH.

Dillman RO (1989) Monoclonal antibodies for treating cancer. Annals of Internal Medicine 111: 592–603.

Dillman RO (2002) Radiolabeled anti-CD20 monoclonal antibodies for the treatment of B-cell lymphoma. Journal of Clinical Oncology 20: 3545–3557.

Draper G, Little M, Sorahan T et al. (1997) Cancer in the offspring of radiation workers: a record linkage study. British Medical Journal 315: 1181–1188.

Effros RB (2003) Genetic alterations in the ageing immune system: impact on infection and cancer. Mechanisms of Ageing and Development 124: 71–77.

Ehrke MJ (2003) Immunomodulation in cancer therapeutics. International Immunopharmacology 451: 1–15.

Entwistle V, Tritter J, Calnan M (2002) Researching experiences of cancer: the importance of methodology. European Journal of Cancer Care 11: 232–237.

ESMO (2001) Minimum clinical recommendations for diagnosis, treatment and follow-up of ovarian cancer. Annals of Oncology 12(9): 1205–1207.

EU Directive 2001/20/EC The Medicines for Human Use (Clinical Trials) Regulations 2003.

European Group for Tumor Markers (EGTM) (1999) Consensus recommendations. Anticancer Res. 19: 2785–820. http://egtm. web.uni-muenchen.de/index2.html; accessed Oct 2002).

Evans D, Evans M (1996) A Decent Proposal: Ethical review of clinical research. Chichester: Wiley.

Fallowfield L (1990) Quality of Life: The missing measurement in health care. London: Souvenir Press.

Fertig DL, Hayes DF (2001) Considerations in using tumour markers: what the psycho-oncologist needs to know. Psycho-Oncology 10: 370–379.

Fielding J, Phenow K (1988) Health effects of involuntary smoking. New England Journal of Medicine 319: 1452–1460.

Fleisher M, Dnistrian AM, Sturgeon CM, Lamerz R, Wittliff JL (2002) Practice guidelines and recommendations for use of tumor markers in the clinic. In: Diamandis EP, Fritsche H, Schwartz MK, Chan DW (eds), Tumor Markers: Physiology, pathobiology, technology and clinical applications. Chicago: AACC Press, pp. 33–63.

Folkman J, Browder T, Palmblad J (2001) Angiogenesis research: guidelines for translation to clinical application. Thrombosis and Haemostasis 8: 23–33.

Foran JM (2002) Antibody-based therapy of non-Hodgkin's lymphoma. Best Practice and Research in Clinical Haematology 15: 449-465.

Fracasso G, Bellisola G, Cingarlini S et al. (2002) Anti-tumour effects of toxins targeted to the prostate specific membrane antigen. The Prostate 53: 9-23.

Franceschi C, Bonafe M, Valensin S (2000) Human immunosenescence: the prevailing of innate immunity, the failing of colotypic immunity, and the filling of immunological space. Vaccine 18: 1717-1720.

Frauwirth KA, Thompson CB (2002) Activation and inhibition of lymphocytes by co-stimulation. Journal of Clinical Investigation 109: 295-299.

Freebairn AJE, Last ATJ, Illidge TM (2001) Trastuzumab: designer drug or fashionable fad? Clinical Oncology 13: 427-433.

Gabriel J (2001) Cancer: health promotion, early detection and staging. In: Gabriel J (ed.), Oncology Nursing in Practice. London: Whurr Publishers.

Gillis C (1978) The epidemiology of human cancers. In: Pritchard P (ed.), Oncology for Nurses and Health Care Professionals. Vol 1, Pathology, Diagnosis and Treatment. London: Harper & Row.

Ginaldi L, Loreta MF, Corsi MP, Modesti M, De Martinis M (2001) Immunosenescence and infectious diseases. Microbes and Infection 3: 851-857.

Glaser B, Strauss A (1967) The Discovery of Grounded Theory: Strategies for qualitative research. New York: Aldine.

Glover D (1999) Fully human monoclonal antibodies come to fruition. Scrip Magazine May: 16-19.

Goldberg D, Williams P (1988) A User's Guide to the General Health Questionnaire. Windsor: NFER-Nelson.

Goodin RE (1995) Utility and the good. In: Singer P (ed.), A Companion to Ethics. Oxford: Blackwell.

Graham J, Ramirez A, Love S, Richards M, Burgess C (2002) Stressful life experiences and risk of relapse of breast cancer: Observational cohort study. British Medical Journal 324: 1420.

Green MC, Murray JL, Hortobagi GN (2000) Monoclonal antibody therapy of solid tumours. Cancer Treatment Reviews 26: 269-286.

Greenhalgh T (2001) How to Read a Paper: The basics of evidence based medicine. London: BMJ Books.

Gulbahce HE, Brown CA, Wick M, Segall M, Jessurun J (2003) Graft-vs-host disease after organ transplant. American Journal of Clinical Pathology 119: 568-573.

Gura T (2002) Magic bullets hit the target. Nature 417: 584-586.

Gusella JF, MacDonald ME (1993) Hunting for Huntington's disease. Molecular Genetics Medicine 3: 139-58.

Hainsworth JD (2000) Monoclonal antibody therapy in lymphoid malignancies. The Oncologist 5: 376-384.

Hait WN (2001) The prognostic and predictive values of ECD-HER-2. Clinical Cancer Research 7: 2601-2604.

Halloran CM, Ghaneh P, Neoptolemos JP, Costello E (2000) Gene therapy for pancreatic cancer - current and prospective strategies. Surgical Oncology 9: 181-191.

Hammersley M, Atkinson P (1983) Ethnography: Principles and practice. London: Tavistock.

Hammond ME, Taube SE (2002) Issues and barriers to development of clinically useful tumor markers: a development pathway proposal. Seminars in Oncology 29: 213-221.

Hammond ME, Fitzgibbons PL, Compton CC et al. (2000) College of American Pathologists Conference XXXV: solid tumor prognostic factors - which, how and so what? Summary document and recommendations for implementation. Cancer Committee and Conference Participants. Archives of Pathology and Laboratory Medicine 124: 958-965 (Review).

Hanahan D, Folkman J (1996) Patterns and emerging mechanisms of the angiogenic switch during tumorigenesis. Cell 86: 353-364.

Hanahan D, Weinberg RA (2000) The hallmarks of cancer. Cell 100: 57-70.

Harries M, Smith I (2002) The development and clinical use of trastuzumab (Herceptin). Endocrine-Related Cancer 9: 75-85.

Harrocopus C, Myers C (eds) (1996) Stoma Care Nursing. London: Edward Arnold.

Hausen L (1991) Viruses in human cancers. Science 254: 1167-1173.

Hayes DF, Trock B, Harris AL (1998) Assessing the clinical impact of prognostic factors: When is 'statistically significant' clinical useful? Breast Cancer Research and Treatment 52: 305-319.

Henson DE, Fielding LP, Grignon DJ et al. (1995) College of American Pathologists Conference XXVI on clinical relevance of prognostic markers in solid tumors. Summary. Archives of Pathology Laboratory Medicine.

Hermansson M, Nist RM, Betsholtz C, Heldin CH, Westermark B, Funa K (1988) Endothelial cell hyperplasia in human glioblastoma: coexpression of mRNA for platelet-derived growth factor (PDGF) B chain and PDGF receptor suggests autocrine growth stimulation. Proceedings of the National Academy of Sciences of the USA 85: 7748-7752.

Holt LJ, Enever C, de Wildt RMT, Tomlinson IM (2000) The use of recombinant antibodies in proteomics. Current Opinion in Biotechnology 11: 445-449.

Hood LE (2003) Chemotherapy in the elderly: supportive measures for chemotherapy-induced myelotoxicity. Clinical Journal of Oncology Nursing 7: 185-190.

Horton-Taylor D (2001) Cancer and epidemiology. In: Corner J, Bailey C (eds), Cancer Nursing: Care in context. Oxford: Blackwell Scientific.

Hudson PJ, Souriau C (1993) Engineered antibodies. Nature Medicine 9: 129-134.

Jenkins V, Fallowfield L (2000) Reasons for accepting or declining to participate in randomised clinical trials for cancer therapy. British Journal of Cancer 82: 1783-1788.

Jorde LB, Carey JC, Bamshad MJ, White RL (2000) Cancer genetics. In: Schmitt W (ed.), Medical Genetics, 2nd edn. St Louis: Mosby, pp. 221-238.

Juweid ME (2002) Radioimmunotherapy of B-cell non-Hodgkin's lymphoma: from clinical trials to clinical practice. Journal of Nuclear Medicine 43: 1507-1529.

Kallioniemi A, Kallioniemi OP, Sudar D et al. (1992) Comparative genomic hybridisation for molecular cytogenetic analysis of solid tumours. Science 258: 818-821.

Kennedy I, Grubb A (2000) Medical Law, 3rd edn. London: Butterworths.

Kerbel R, Folkman J (2002) Clinical translation of angiogenesis inhibitors. Nature Review of Cancer 2: 727-739.

Ketcham M, Loescher L (2000) Skin cancers. In: Greonwald S, Frogge M, Goodman M, Yarbro C (eds), Cancer Nursing: Principles and practice. Boston, MA: Jones & Bartlett.

Kinzler KW, Vogelstein B (1996) Lessons from hereditary colorectal cancer. Cell 87: 159-170.

Kirkbride KC, Blobe GC (2003) Inhibition of the TGFβ signalling pathway as means of cancer immunotherapy. Expert Opinion Biological Therapy 3: 251-261.

Klapdor R, Aronsson AC, Duffy MJ et al. (1999) Tumor markers in gastrointestinal cancers: EGTM recommendations. Anticancer Research 19: 2811-2815.

Knudson AG Jr (1971) Mutation and cancer: statistical study of retinoblastoma. Proceedings of the National Academy of Sciences of the USA 68: 820-823.

Koch T (1995) Interpretive approaches in nursing research: the influence of Husserl and Heidegger. Journal of Advanced Nursing 24: 827–836.

Koch T (1996) Implementation of a hermeneutic inquiry in nursing: philosophy, rigour and representation. Journal of Advanced Nursing 24: 174–184.

Köhler G, Milstein C (1975) Continuous culture of fused cells secreting specific antibody of predefined specificity. Nature 256: 495–497.

Kricka LJ (2000) Interferences in immunoassay – still a threat [Editorial]. Clinical Chemistry 46: 1037–1038.

Kubota Y, Ohji H, Itoh K, Sasagawa I, Nakada T (2001). Changes in cellular immunity during chemotherapy for testicular cancer. International Journal of Urology 8: 604–608.

Kuroki M, Ueno A, Mastumoto H et al. (2002). Significance of tumour-associated antigens in the diagnosis and therapy of cancer: an overview. Anticancer Research 22: 4255–4264.

Kyle RA (1975) Multiple myeloma: review of 869 cases. Mayo Clinic Proceedings 50: 29–40.

Lal A, Lash AE, Altschul SF et al. (1999) A public database for gene expression in human cancers. Cancer Research 59: 5403–5407.

Lamerz R, Albrecht W, Bialk P, et al. (1999) Tumour markers in germ cell cancers: EGTM recommendations. Anticancer Research 19: 2795–2798.

Leitner WW, Ying H, Restifo NP (2000) DNA and RNA-based vaccines: principles, progress and prospects (Review). Vaccines 18: 765–777.

LeMarbre P, Greonwald S (2000) Biology of cancer. In: Greonwald S, Frogge M, Goodman M, Yarbro C (eds), Cancer Nursing: Principles and practice. Boston, MA: Jones & Bartlett.

Leonard JP, Link BK (2002) Immunotherapy of non-Hodgkin's lymphoma with hLL2 (Epratuzumab, an anti-CD-22 monoclonal antibody) and HUD10 (Apolizumab). Seminars in Oncology 29(suppl 2): 81–86.

Levings MK, Bacchetta R, Schultz U, Roncarolo MG (2002) The role of IL-10 and TGF-beta in the differentiation and effector function of T regulatory cells. International Archives of Allergy and Immunology 129: 263–276.

Lewin B (1994) Genes V. Oxford: Oxford University Press.

Lewin B (2000) Genes VII. Oxford: Oxford University Press.

Ligibel JA, Winer EP (2002) Trastuzumab/chemotherapy combinations in metastatic breast cancer. Seminars in Oncology 29(suppl 11): 38–43.

Lind J, Hagan L (1997) Bladder and kidney cancer. In: Greonwald S, Frogge M, Goodman M, Yarbro C (eds), Cancer Nursing: Principles and practice. Boston, MA: Jones & Bartlett.

LoBiondo-Wood G, Haber J (1998) Nursing Research: Methods, critical appraisal, and utilization, 4th edn. London: Mosby.

Loeb LA (1994) Microsatellite instability: marker of a mutator phenotype in cancer. Cancer Research 54: 5059–5063.

Lollini PL, Forni G (2003) Cancer immunoprevention: tracking down persistent tumour antigens. Trends in Immunology 24(2): 62–66.

Lords JM, Butcher S, Killampali V, Lascelles D, Salmon M (2001) Neutrophil ageing and immunesence. Mechanisms of Ageing and Development 122: 1521–1535.

Lundqvist A, Pisa P (2002) Gene-modified dendritic cells and immunotherapy against cancer. Medical Oncology 19: 197–211

Lutz J, Heemann U (2003) Tumours after kidney transplantation. Current Opinion in Urology 13: 105–109.

Lynch H, Alban W (1984) Genetic biomarkers and the Heieck control of breast cancer. Cancer Genetics and Cytogenetics 13: 43–92.

McHugh RS, Shevach EM (2002) The role of suppressor T cells in regulation of immune responses. Allergy and Clinical Immunology 110: 693-702.

Macleod K (2000) Tumor suppressor genes. Current Opinion in Genetic Development 10: 81-93.

Madsen S et al. (2002) Attitudes towards clinical trials. Journal of Internal Medicine 251: 156-168.

Magdelenat H (1992) Tumour markers in oncology: past, present and future. Journal of Immunological Methods 150: 133-143.

Malaguaranera L, Ferlito L, Di Mauro S, Imbesi RM, Scalia G, Malaguarnero M (2001) Immunosenescence and cancer: a review. Archives of Gerontology and Geriatrics 32(2): 77-93.

Marks C, Marks JD (1996). Phage libraries: A new route to clinically useful antibodies. New England Journal of Medicine 335: 730-733.

Marks V (2002) False-positive immunoassay results: A multicenter survey of erroneous immunoassay results from assays of 74 analytes in 10 donors from 66 laboratories in seven countries. Clinical Chemistry.

Mays N, Pope C (1995) Qualitative research: rigour and qualitative research. British Medical Journal 311: 109-112

Mendelsohn J (2001) The epidermal growth factor receptor as a target for cancer therapy. Endocrine-related Cancer 8: 3-9.

Miles LE, Hales CN (1968a) Immunoradiometric assay of human growth hormone. Lancet ii: 492-493.

Miles LEH, Hales CN (1968b) Labelled antibodies and immunological assay systems. Nature 219: 186-189.

Miller RA (1996) The ageing immune system: primer and prospectus. Science 273: 70-74.

Modjtahedi H, Dean C (1994) The receptor for EGF and its ligands: expression, prognostic value and target for therapy in cancer (Review). International Journal of Oncology 4: 277-296.

Modjtahedi H, Hickish T, Nicolson M et al. (1996). A phase I trial and tumour localisation of the anti-EGFR antibody ICR62 in head and neck or lung cancer. British Journal of Cancer 73: 228-235.

Moingeon P (2001) Cancer vaccines (review). Vaccine 19: 1305-1326.

Molina R, Duffy MJ, Aronsson AC et al. (1999) Tumor markers in breast cancer: EGTM recommendations. Anticancer Research 19: 2803-2805.

Morimoto Y, Tanaka Y, Itoh T, Yamamoto S, Mizuno H, Fushimi H (2002) Spontaneous necrosis of hepatocellular carcinoma: a case report. Digestive Surgery 19: 413-418.

Munhall P (1982) Nursing philosophy and nursing research: in apposition or opposition. Nursing Research 31: 176-177.

Naito Y, Saito K, Shiiba K et al. (1998) CD8+ T cells infiltrated within cancer cell nests as a prognostic factor in human colorectal cancer. Cancer Research 58: 3491-3494.

Nakano O, Sato M, Naito Y et al. (2001) Proliferation activity of intratumoural CD8+ T-lymphocytes as a prognostic factor in human renal cell carcinoma: clinicopathogenic demonstration of antitumour immunity. Cancer Research 61: 5132-5136.

Nakayama Y, Nagashima N, Minagawa N et al. (2002). Relationship between tumor associated macrophages and clinicopathological factors in patients with colorectal cancer. Anticancer Research 22: 4291-4296.

Natali PG, Nicotra MR, Bigotti A et al. (1989) Selective changes in expression of HLA class I polymorphic determinants in human tumours. Proceedings of the National Academy Sciences of the USA 86: 6719-6723.

National Cancer Research Network (2001) Newsletter, November.

National Translational Cancer Research Network (2002) Mission Statement (www.ntrac.org.uk; accessed 17 Feb 2003)

Needle MN (2002) Safety experience with IMC-225, an anti-epidermal growth factor receptor antibody. Seminars in Oncology 29(suppl 14): 55-60.

Nicholson RI, Gee JMW, Harper ME (2001) EGFR and cancer prognosis. European Journal of Cancer 37: S9-S15.

Nursing and Midwifery Council (NMC) (2000) Research and Audit. London: NMC.

NMC (2002) Code of Professional Conduct. London: NMC.

Nustad K, Bast RC Jr, Brien TJ et al. (1996) Specificity and affinity of 26 monoclonal antibodies against the CA 125 antigen: first report from the ISOBM TD-1 workshop. International Society for Oncodevelopmental Biology and Medicine. Tumour Biology 17: 196-219.

O'Mahony M (2001) Women's lived experience of breast biopsy: a phenomenological study. Journal of Clinical Nursing 10: 512-520.

O'Mary S (2000) Diagnostic evaluation, classification and staging. In: Greonwald S, Frogge M, Goodman M, Yarbro C (eds), Cancer Nursing: Principles and practice. Boston, MA: Jones & Bartlett.

O'Neill O (1995) Kantian ethics. In: Singer P (ed.), A Companion to Ethics. Oxford: Blackwell.

Ohno S, Inagawa H, Soma GI, Nagasue N (2002) Role of tumour-associated macrophages in malignant tumours: should the location of the infiltrated macrophages be taken into account during evaluation? Anticancer Research 22: 4269-4276.

Pagliargo LC, Liu B, Munker R et al. (1998) Humanized M195 monoclonal antibody conjugate to recombinant Gelonin: an anti-CD33 immunotoxin with antileukemic activity. Clinical Cancer Research 4: 1971-1976.

Paley J (1997) Husserl, phenomenology and nursing. Journal of Advanced Nursing 26: 187-193.

Palmer A (2001) Understanding radiotherapy and its applications. In: Gabriel J (ed.), Oncology Nursing in Practice. London: Whurr.

Pangalis GA, Dimopoulou MN, Angelopoulou MK et al. (2001) Campath-1H (Anti-CD520 monoclonal antibody therapy in lymphoproliferative disorders. Medical Oncology 18: 99-107.

Papac RJ (1998) Spontaneous regression of cancer: possible mechanisms. In Vivo 12: 571-578.

Parahoo K (1997) Nursing Research: Principles, process and issues. London: Macmillan.

Pardoll DM (1998) Cancer vaccines. Nature Medicine 4 (Suppl 5): 525-531.

Paschin A, Mendez RM, Jimenez P et al. (2003) Complete loss of HLA Class I antigen expression on melanoma cells: a result of successive mutational events. International Journal of Cancer 103: 759-769.

Pinedo H, Salmon D (2000) Translational Research. The role of VEGF in tumour angiogenesis. The Oncologist (supp1): 1-2.

Ponder BA (2001) Cancer genetics. Nature 411: 336-341.

Popay J, Williams G (1998) Qualitative research and evidence-based healthcare Journal of the Royal Society of Medicine 91(35): 32-37.

Price B (1990) Body Image: Nursing concepts and care. London: Prentice Hall.

Rai KR, Freter CE, Mercier RJ et al. (2002) Alemtuzumab in previously treated chronic lymphocytic leukemia patients who also received fludarabine. Journal of Clinical Oncology 20: 3891-3897.

Ramirez A, Craig T, Watson J, Fentiman I, North W, Rubens R (1989) Stress and relapse of breast cancer. British Medical Journal 298: 291-293.

Ray-Coquard I, Borg C, Bachelot T et al. for the ELYPSE study group (2003) Baseline and early lymphopenia predict for the risk of febrile neutropenia after chemotherapy. British Journal of Cancer 88: 181-186.

Reeves G, Todd I (2000) Lecture notes on Immunology. London: Blackwell Science.

Reik W, Walter J (2001) Genomic imprinting: parental influence on the genome. Nature Review of Genetics 2: 21-32.

Rhee I, Jair KW, Yen RW et al. (2000) CpG methylation is maintained in human cancer cells lacking DNMT1. Nature 404: 1003-1007.

Richards TI, Richards L (1990) Manual for Mainframe NUD.IST Software Version 2.1. Melbourne: Replee.

Richardson A, Miller M, Potter H (2002) Developing, Delivering and Evaluating Cancer Nursing Services: Building the evidence base. London: King's College.

Romero P, Pittet M, Dutoit V et al. (2002) Therapeutic cancer vaccines based on molecularly defined human tumour antigens. Vaccine 20: A2-A7.

Ropponen KM, Eskelinen MJ, Lipponen PK, Alhava E, Kosma VM (1997) Prognostic value of tumour infiltrating lymphocytes (TILs) in colorectal cancer. Journal of Pathology 182: 318-324.

Royal College of Radiologists' Clinical Oncology Information Network and British Association of Urological Surgeons (1999) Guidelines on the management of prostate cancer. A document for local expert groups in the United Kingdom preparing prostate management policy documents. BJU International 84: 987-1014.

Rubin I, Yarden Y (2001) The basic biology of HER-2. Annals on Oncology 12(suppl 1): S3-S8.

Sabel MS, Sondak VK (2002). Melanoma vaccines: breakthrough or bust? Cancer Investigation 20: 1114-1116.

Salgaller ML, Tjoa BA, Lodge PA et al. (1998) Dendritic cell-based immunotherapy of prostate cancer. Critical Review. Immunology 18: 109-119.

Salkind N (2000) Statistics for People Who Hate Statistics. London: Sage.

Scadden DT (2003) AIDS-related malignancies. Annual Review of Medicine 54: 285-303.

Schilsky RL, Taube SE (2002) Tumor markers as clinical cancer tests - are we there yet? Seminars in Oncology 29: 211-212.

Scott SD (1998) Rituximab: A new therapeutic monoclonal antibody for non-Hodgkin's lymphoma. Cancer Practice 6: 195-197.

Sell S (1991) Cancer markers. In: Mossa AR, Scimpff SC, Roboson (eds), Comprehensive Textbook of Oncology. Baltimore, MA: Williams & Wilkins, pp. 225-238.

Semjonow A, Albrecht W, Bialk P et al. (1999) Tumour markers in prostate cancer: EGTM recommendations. Anticancer Research 19: 2799-2801.

Sheppard C (2001) Breast cancer. In: Gabriel J (ed.), Oncology Nursing in Practice. London: Whurr.

Shimada H, Ochiai T, Nomura F (2003) Titration of serum p53 antibodies in 1085 patients with various types of malignant tumours. Cancer 97: 682-689.

Sliwkowski MX, Lofgren JA, Lewis GD, Hotaling TE, Fendly BM, Fox J (1999) Nonclinical studies addressing the mechanism of action of trastuzumab (Herceptin). Seminars in Oncology 26(suppl 12): 60-70.

Solana R, Mariani E (2000) NK and NK/T cells in human senescence. Vaccine 18: 1613-1620.

Southern EM (1975) Detection of specific sequences among DNA fragments separated by gel electrophoresis. Journal of Molecular Biology 98: 503-517.

Sporn MB (1996) The war on cancer. Lancet 347: 1377-81.

Sprangers M, Cull A, Bjordal K, Groenvold M, Aaronson N (1993) The European Organization for Research and Treatment of Cancer approach to quality of life assessment: guidelines for developing questionnaire modules. Quality of Life Research 2: 287-295.

Sprent J (2003) Turnover of memory-phenotype CD8+ T cells. Microbes and Infection 5: 227-231.

Sprent J, Surh CD (2003) Cytokines and T-cell homeostasis. Immunology Letters 85: 145-149.

Stacy S, Krolick KA, Infante AJ, Kraig E (2002) Immunological memory and late onset autoimmunity. Mechanisms of Ageing and Development 123: 975-985.

Stenman UH, Paus E, Allard WJ et al. (1999) Summary report of the TD-3 workshop: characterization of 83 antibodies against prostate-specific antigen. Tumour Biology 2(suppl 1): 1-12

Stieber P, Aronsson AC, Bialk P et al. (1999) Tumor markers in lung cancer: EGTM recommendations. Anticancer Research 19: 2817-2819.

Strachan T, Read AP (1999) DNA structure and gene expression. In: Human Molecular Genetics 2. Oxford: BIOS Scientific Publishers.

Strausberg RL (2001) The Cancer Genome Anatomy Project: new resources for reading the molecular signatures of cancer. Journal of Pathology 195: 31-40 (review).

Strausberg RL, Dahl CA, Klausner RD (1997) New opportunities for uncovering the molecular basis of cancer. Nature Genetics 15: 415-416.

Strausberg RL, Buetow KH, Emmert-Buck MR, Klausner RD (2000)The cancer genome anatomy project: building an annotated gene index. Trends in Genetics 16: 103-106.

Strausberg RL, Camargo AA, Riggins GJ et al. (2002) An international database and integrated analysis tools for the study of cancer gene expression. Pharmacogenomics Journal 2: 156-164.

Strausberg RL, Simpson AJ, Wooster R (2003) Sequence-based cancer genomics: progress, lessons and opportunities. National Review of Genetics 4(6): 409-418.

Strauss and Corbin (1990) Basics of Qualitative Research: Grounded theory, procedures and techniques. Thousand Oaks, CA: Sage.

Sturgeon CM (2001) Tumor markers in the laboratory: closing the guideline-practice gap. Clinical Biochemistry 34: 353-359.

Sturgeon C (2002) Practice guidelines for tumor maker use in the clinic. Clinical Chemistry 48: 1151-1159.

Sturgeon CM, Seth J (1996) Why do immunoassays for tumour markers give differing results? – A view from the UK National External Quality Assessment Schemes. European Journal of Clinical Chemistry and Biochemistry 34: 755-759.

Sturgeon C, Aronsson AC, Duffy MJ, Hansson LO, Klapdor R, Van Dalen A (1999a) European Group of Tumour Markers: Consensus recommendations. Anticancer Research 19: 2785-2820.

Sturgeon C, Dati F, Duffy MJ et al. (1999b) Quality requirements and control: EGTM recommendations. Anticancer Research 19: 2791-2794.

Suresh MR (2001) Cancer marker. In: Wild D (ed) The Immunoassay Handbook, 2nd edn. Nature Publishing Group, pp. 635-663.

Sweep CG, Geurts-Moespot J (2000) EORT external quality assurance program for ER and PgR measurements: trial 1998/1999. European Organisation for Research and Treatment of Cancer. Internal Journal of Biological Markers 15(1): 62–69.

Tagawa M (2000) Cytokine therapy for cancer. Cancer Pharmaceutical Design 6: 681–699.

Thibodeau J, MacRae J (1997) Breast cancer survival: A phenomenological inquiry. Advanced Nursing Science 19(4): 65–74.

Thomas CMG, Sweep CGJ (2001) Serum tumour markers: past, state of art and future. International Journal of Biological Markers 16(2): 73–85.

Thomas J, Retsas A (1999) Transacting self preservation: a grounded theory of the spiritual dimensions of people with terminal cancer. International Journal of Nursing Studies 36: 191–201.

Tjoa BA, Erickson SJ, Bowes VA et al. (1997) Follow-up evaluation of prostate cancer patients infused with autologous dendritic cells pulsed with PSMA peptides. The Prostate 32: 272–278.

Tortora GJ, Grabowski SR (2003) Principles of Anatomy and Physiology, 10th edn. New York: Harper Collins/Addison Wesley, pp. 764–804.

Trask BJ (1991) Fluorescence in situ hybridization: applications in cytogenetics and gene mapping. Trends in Genetics 7: 149–154.

Tumor Marker Expert Panel (ASCO) (1996) Clinical practice guidelines for the use of tumor markers in breast and colorectal cancer. Journal of Clinical Oncology 14: 2843–2877.

UICC (International Union Against Cancer) (1997) TNM Classification of Malignant Tumours (5th edition) New York: Wiley-Liss.

Valley AW (2002) New treatment options for managing chemotherapy-induced neutropenia. American Journal Health-System Pharmacy 59(15)(suppl 4): S11–S16.

Van der Zalm J, Bergum V (2000) Hermeneutic–phenomenology: providing living knowledge for nursing practice. Journal of Advanced Nursing 31(1): 211–218.

Van Manen M (1990) Researching Lived Experience: Human science for an action sensitive pedagogy. New York: State University of New York Press.

Venitt S (1978) The aetiology of human cancers. In: Pritchard P (ed.), Oncology for Nurses and Health Care Professionals. Vol 1, Pathology, Diagnosis and Treatment. London: Harper & Row.

Vial T, Descotes J (2003) Immunosuppressive drugs and cancer. Toxicology 185: 229–240.

Voet D, Voet JG (1995) The expression and transmission of genetic information. In: Biochemistry. New York: John Wiley & Sons.

Waldman H (2002) A personal history of Campath-1H antibody. Medical Oncology 19: S3–S9.

Waldman TA (2003) Immunotherapy: past, present and future. Nature Medicine 9: 269–277.

Waldman TA (2003) Immunotherapy: past, present and future. Nature Medicine 9: 269–277.

Walker RA (2000) The significance of histological determination of HER-2 status in breast cancer. The Breast 9: 130–133.

Walter J (1977) Radiation hazards and protection: Cytotoxic chemotherapy. In: Walter J (ed.), Cancer and Radiotherapy: A short guide for nurses and medical students. London: Churchill Livingstone.

Ward RL, Hawkins NJ, Smith GM (1997) Unconjugated antibodies for cancer therapy: lessons from the clinic. Cancer Treatment Reviews 23: 305–319.

Watson JD, Crick FHC (1953) Molecular study of nucleic acids. Nature 171: 737–738.

Webb N, Bottomley M, Watson C, Brenchley P (1998) Vascular endothelial growth factor (VEGF) is released from platelets during blood clotting: implications for measurement of circulating VEGF levels in clinical disease. Clinical Science 94: 395–404.

Westgard JO, Barry PL (1986) Improving quality control by use of multirule control procedures. In: Cost-Effective Quality Control: Managing the quality and productivity of analytical processes. Washington, DC: AACC Press, pp. 92–117.

Westgard JO, Barry PL, Hunt MR, Groth T (1981) A multi-rule Shewhart chart for quality control in clinical chemistry. Clinical Chemistry 27: 493–501.

Whittaker J, Sheppard C (2001) Body image and sexuality. In: Gabriel J (ed.), Oncology Nursing in Practice. London: Whurr Publishers.

Willett W (1989) The search for the cause of breast and colon cancer. Nature 338: 389–394.

Williams JG, Ceccarelli A, Spurr N (1995) Gene organisation and expression. In: Williams J, Ceccarelli A, Wallace A (eds) Genetic Engineering. Oxford: BIOS Scientific.

Wimpenny P, Gass J (2000) Interviewing in phenomenology and grounded theory: is there a difference? Journal of Advanced Nursing 31: 1485–1492.

Winter G, Milstein C (1991) Man-made antibodies. Nature 349: 293–299.

Wolfe N (1986) Neoplasia: Disorders of cell proliferation and differentiation. In: Cell, Tissue and Disease: The basis of pathology. London: Baillière Tindall.

Wood P (2001) Understanding Immunology. Harlow: Prentice Hall.

Workman P, Kaye S (2002) Translating basic cancer research into new cancer therapies. Trends in Molecular Medicine 8: S1–S9.

Xiao W, Oefner PJ (2001) Denaturing high-performance liquid chromatography: A review. Human Mutations 17: 439–474.

Yalow RS, Berson SA (1960) Immunoassay of endogenous plasma insulin in man. Journal of Clinical Investigation 39: 1157–1175.

Yang XD, Jia XC, Corvalan JRF, Wang P, Deavis G (2001) Development of ABX-EGF, a fully human anti-EGF receptor monoclonal antibody, for cancer therapy. Critical Reviews in Oncology/Hematology 38: 17–23.

Yao D, Trabulsi EJ, Kostakoglu L et al. (2002) Seminars in Urologic Oncology 20: 211–218.

Yarbro J (2000a) Milestones in our understanding of cancer. In: Greonwald,S, Frogge M, Goodman M, Yarbro C (eds), Cancer Nursing: Principles and practice. Boston, MA: Jones & Bartlett.

Yarbro J (2000b) Carcinogensis. In: Greonwald S, Frogge M, Goodman M, Yarbro C (eds), Cancer Nursing: Principles and practice. Boston, MA: Jones & Bartlett.

Young CD, Feld R (2000) Approaches to the management of infections in cancer patients with neutropenia. In: Cavalli F, Hansen HH, Kaye SB (eds), Textbook of Medical Oncology. London: Martin Dunitz, pp. 565–581.

Young W (2001) Breaking bad news. In: Gabriel J (ed.), Oncology Nursing in Practice. London: Whurr Publishers.

Zigmond A, Snaith R (1983) The Hospital Anxiety and Depression Scale. Acta Psychiatrica Scandinavica 67: 361–370.

Index

DNA polymerase, 54
DNA-repair genes, 67
docetaxel, 47
dominant genetic disorders, 62
doxorubicin, 45, 48
Duchenne muscular dystrophy, 61–62
Dukes' staging system, 7
dynamic tumour markers, 99
dysplastic naevus syndrome, 17

E2F family, 38, 39
early detection, 20–21
E-cadherin, 43
endocrine glands, 40
endoplasmic reticulum (ER), 34–35
endoscopy, 10
enhancer elements, 59
enzyme-linked immunosorbent assay
     (ELISA/EIA), 101
EORTC Quality of Life Questionnaire,
     141
epidermal growth factor receptor
     (EGFR), 117
epithelia and epithelial cells, 40, 41
epratuzumab, 119
Epstein–Barr virus, 15
erythrocytes, 41
Escherichia coli, 53
ethical issues, research, 156–159
     participant, 166–169
     research, 164–166
     researcher, 159–164
ethnography, 153–154
etoposide, 47, 49
eukaryotes, 33–35, 56
European Convention on Human
     Rights, 158
European Group for Tumor Markers
     (EGTM), 104
exercise, 19
exocrine glands, 40
exocytosis, 81
exons, 56, 59, 60
extracellular pathogens, 76

FACC gene, 17
faecal occult blood test, 20
familial adenomatous polyposis (FAP),
     72
familial hypercholesterolaemia, 73
familial polyposis, 17

Fanconi's anaemia, 17
fats, dietary, 12, 13
febrile neutropenia, 94
fibre, dietary, 12, 13
fibroblasts, 40
filgrastim, 95
flexible sigmoidoscopy, 20
fluorescence in situ hybridization
     (FISH), 69–70, 101
5-fluorouracil (5FU), 46, 49
frameshift effect, 61, 62
Franklin, Rosalind, 52
French, American and British (FAB)
     classifications, 7
Functional Assessment of Cancer
     Therapy, 141

gamma camera, 9
gamma rays, 8
gap 0 (G0), 36
gap 1 (G1), 36, 38, 39
gap 2 (G2), 36, 38
gastric cancer, 5, 13, 15, 67
GC suppression, 68
gemtuzumab ozogamicin (Mylotarg),
     115, 123–124
gene chips, 96, 107
General Health Questionnaire, 141
genes and genetics
     defining chromosomal
          abnormalities in a tumour,
          69–70
     DNA-repair genes, 67
     future applications, 72–73
     gene therapy, 72–73, 129
     genetic disease, 61–65
     identifying cancer genes, 69
     insertions and deletions, 61
     methylation in tumorigenesis,
          67–69
     mutations, 59–60
          analysis, 70–71
     nature of, 59
     oncogenes, 65
     as predisposing factor, 17
     research, 28
     screening for cancer, 71–72
     single base substitutions, 60–61
     translocations, 133
     tumour suppressor genes, 65–67
     see also DNA